PRAISE FOR *CARITAS COACHING*

"*An intimate window into the most personal journey of Caritas Coaches as they infuse their lives and practice with Caring Science, transforming their capacity to extend the same unconditional loving kindness to their fellow spirit-filled beings. A significant contribution to advancing caritas literacy.*"

–Jacqueline G. Somerville, PhD, RN, FAAN
Chief Nurse Executive, The Hospital of the University of Pennsylvania
Certified Caritas Coach

"*The demands on caring professionals are ever-increasing, and as a result, there is an epidemic of stress, anxiety, and burnout. The integration of the practices outlined in the Caritas Coach Education Program (CCEP) are transformational. Caritas Coaching not only shares such stories of transformation but also provides a road map of how each of us in the caring profession can care for ourselves and, by doing so, be better caregivers.*"

–James R. Doty, MD
Professor of Neurosurgery and Founder and Director
Center for Compassion and Altruism Research and Education,
Stanford University School of Medicine

"*Sara Horton-Deutsch and Jan Anderson have created a road map for a transformational journey to a personal life and professional nursing practice that reflect the deep wisdom embodied in Caring Science. Embrace this wisdom, embark on this journey, and be the change that you want to see in nursing and healthcare.*"

–Marlaine C. Smith, PhD, RN, AHN-BC, FAAN
Dean and Helen K. Persson Eminent Scholar
Christine E. Lynn College of Nursing
Florida Atlantic University

"Caritas Coaching *opens the mind, soul, and spirit to a deeper and more meaningful understanding of health. Our journey with self and other—as partners in sharing our story and their stories about the personal and intimate spaces we find and nurture in life—is amplified in a beautiful and vibrant frequency in this work by Horton-Deutsch and Anderson. Truly a work of healing ourselves as we move forward in our practice of caring for others with the heart and mind—the most beautiful blend of artistry and science.*"

–Neal Rosenburg, PhD, RN
Dean and Professor
College of Health Professions & McAuley School of Nursing, University of Detroit Mercy

"*Horton-Deutsch and Anderson provide a clear and compelling introduction to Watson's Caring Science. The contributors share vivid portraits of transformation that will instruct and inspire newcomers and well-seasoned caritas professionals alike. This book is a must-read for anyone interested in creating and sustaining loving-caring purpose, hope, and joy in professional life and beyond.*"

–Kathleen Sitzman, PhD, RN, CNE, ANEF, FAAN
Professor, East Carolina University College of Nursing

"*This text offers an intimate narrative of what it truly means to pursue the path of a Caritas Coach. The authors share insightful learning experiences of reflection, self-discovery, and healing as they advanced through a structured Caritas Coach Education Program. The program is grounded in Jean Watson's 10 Caritas Processes, which give voice to the theory of human caring and serve as a framework for informed moral action by educators, leaders, and practitioners. The outcomes and values of the Caritas Coach program are embodied in its nearly 350 graduates across the globe, whose precious personal stories engender hope through renewed purpose and authentic transformation of self and systems from the inside out.*"

–Jim D'Alfonso, DNP, PhD(h), RN, NEA-BC, FNAP
Founding CNE/COO, Watson Caring Science Institute, Boulder, CO
(2008–2011)
Executive Director, Professional Practice, Leadership Development and Research
Founding Executive Director, Kaiser Permanente's Nurse Scholars Academy
Kaiser Permanente, Oakland, CA

"As a seasoned nurse and healthcare executive, I have been forced at various stages in my career to ask important and difficult questions about the purpose of my work—and whether I am truly modeling the way to a caring and heart-centered practice. Caritas Coaching *is a powerful tool with wonderful storytelling from many perspectives that grounds us in theory and guides us in the sacred work of healthcare.* Caritas Coaching *reminds us of our healer within and the power of supporting an organizational culture of transpersonal caring. For each of us in this difficult work,* Caritas Coaching *provides practical and theory-based resources to achieve professional fulfillment, joy in our work, and the sustained ability for a caring and healing practice."*

–Kelly Johnson, PhD, RN, NEA-BC
Vice President for Patient Care Services and Chief Nursing Officer
Lucile Packard Children's Hospital Stanford
Clinical Associate Professor (Affiliated)
Division of Neurology and Neurosciences
Stanford University School of Medicine

"If you are a Caritas Coach—or simply have a heart's desire to understand, feel, and learn a new way of integrating the depth of our humanity, love, and soul into our practice and evolutionary journey—this book is for you. It will fill you with a wealth of insight from some of the most compelling Caritas Coaches of our time. Horton-Deutsch and Anderson have done an exquisite job of revealing to the world some of the most core aspects of Caring Science and its meaningful applications into the micro aspects of our life through the stories of others."

—Robert Browning, PhD (h.c.)
Director & Senior Trainer, HeartMath
Faculty & Board Member, Watson Caring Science Institute
Co-VP, Pathways to Peace, a UN Peace Messenger Organization with ECOSOC
Consultative Status

Caritas COACHING

A Journey Toward Transpersonal Caring for Informed Moral Action in Healthcare

Sara Horton-Deutsch, PhD, RN, FAAN, ANEF, Caritas Coach
Jan Anderson, EdD, MSN, RN, AHN-BC, Caritas Coach

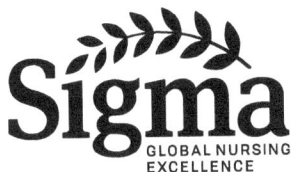

Sigma
GLOBAL NURSING
EXCELLENCE

The Sigma Theta Tau International Honor Society of Nursing (Sigma) is a nonprofit organization whose mission is advancing world health and celebrating nursing excellence in scholarship, leadership, and service. Founded in 1922, Sigma has more than 135,000 active members in over 90 countries and territories. Members include practicing nurses, instructors, researchers, policymakers, entrepreneurs, and others. Sigma's more than 530 chapters are located at more than 700 institutions of higher education throughout Armenia, Australia, Botswana, Brazil, Canada, Colombia, England, Ghana, Hong Kong, Japan, Jordan, Kenya, Lebanon, Malawi, Mexico, the Netherlands, Pakistan, Philippines, Portugal, Singapore, South Africa, South Korea, Swaziland, Sweden, Taiwan, Tanzania, Thailand, the United States, and Wales. Learn more at www.sigmanursing.org.

Sigma Theta Tau International
550 West North Street
Indianapolis, IN, USA 46202

To order additional books, buy in bulk, or order for corporate use, contact Nursing Knowledge International at 888. NKI.4YOU (888.654.4968/US and Canada) or +1.317.634.8171 (outside US and Canada).

To request a review copy for course adoption, email solutions@nursingknowledge.org or call 888.NKI.4YOU (888.654.4968/US and Canada) or +1.317.634.8171 (outside US and Canada).

To request author information, or for speaker or other media requests, contact Marketing, Honor Society of Nursing, Sigma Theta Tau International at 888.634.7575 (US and Canada) or +1.317.634.8171 (outside US and Canada).

ISBN: 9781945157295
EPUB ISBN: 9781945157301
PDF ISBN: 9781945157318
MOBI ISBN: 9781945157325

Library of Congress Cataloging-in-Publication data

Names: Horton-Deutsch, Sara, author. | Anderson, Jan, 1952 January 19- author. | Sigma Theta Tau International, issuing body.
Title: Caritas coaching : a journey toward transpersonal caring for informed moral action in healthcare / Sara Horton-Deutsch, Jan Anderson.
Description: Indianapolis, IN : Sigma Theta Tau International, [2018] | Includes bibliographical references.
Identifiers: LCCN 2017057105 (print) | LCCN 2017060185 (ebook) | ISBN 9781945157301 (Epub) | ISBN 9781945157318 (Pdf) | ISBN 9781945157325 (Mobi) | ISBN 9781945157295 (print : alk. paper) | ISBN 9781945157325 (MOBI)
Subjects: | MESH: Nurse-Patient Relations | Empathy | Self Care | Holistic Nursing | Ethics, Nursing | Interprofessional Relations
Classification: LCC R697.A4 (ebook) | LCC R697.A4 (print) | NLM WY 88 | DDC 610.73/7--dc23
LC record available at https://lccn.loc.gov/2017057105

First Printing, 2018

Publisher: Dustin Sullivan
Acquisitions Editor: Emily Hatch
Editorial Coordinator: Paula Jeffers
Cover Designer: Rebecca Batchelor
Interior Design/Page Layout: Rebecca Batchelor

Principal Book Editor: Carla Hall
Development and Project Editor: Kate Shoup
Copy Editor: Meaghan O'Keeffe
Proofreader: Todd Lothery
Indexer: Larry Sweazy

DEDICATION

These stories of healing are dedicated to healthcare professionals and caregivers around the world who are seeking ways to reclaim the joy and fulfillment of caring for self and other. May they inspire all readers to reconnect with their meaning and purpose in life.

Acknowledgments

We acknowledge with love and appreciation the over 300 Caritas Coaches worldwide who have had the courage to enter this lifelong journey of self-discovery and self-love to find healing and peace.

A special thank you to the vision and wisdom of Dr. Jean Watson, who has inspired nursing and health professionals for more than 40 years, and to those faculty and nursing leaders who have so freely shared their expertise to co-create and to serve as living exemplars of this work.

ABOUT THE AUTHORS

Sara Horton-Deutsch, PhD, RN, FAAN, ANEF, Caritas Coach, is a professor and serves as the Jean Watson Caring Science Endowed Chair at the University of Colorado College of Nursing. Her mission is to advance the art and science of human caring knowledge, ethics, and clinical practice in the fields of nursing and health sciences. Her work fosters research, teaching, and practice of human caring through an interprofessional PhD program and continuing education training programs that integrate new knowledge from humanities, arts, cross-cultural spiritual disciplines, and emerging scientific disciplines. In 2015, Horton-Deutsch also was appointed as an Assistant Director for the Center for Bioethics and Humanities at the University of Colorado-Denver, which assembles colleagues from across the campus, university, state, and nation to support competent, compassionate, and respectful healthcare through teaching, research, clinical service, and community engagement.

Horton-Deutsch's work in reflective practice has been published in two books coedited with Dr. Gwen Sherwood: *Reflective Practice: Transforming Education and Improving Outcomes* (Sigma Theta Tau International, 2012) and *Reflective Organizations: On the Front Lines of QSEN & Reflective Practice Implementation* (Sigma Theta Tau International, 2015). The latter was recognized as 2015 AJN Book of the Year. Clinical nurses and academic programs around the world use these books to support deep learning that leads to intentional, effective, and thoughtful action. It was through the iterative process of reflection that Horton-Deutsch deepened her own work in reflective practice, resulting in the integration of Caring Science. Like reflective practice, Caring Science calls healthcare professionals to actions that honor all living things.

Horton-Deutsch has been an active participant in the Quality and Safety Education for Nurses (QSEN) initiative, contributing to the publication of web-based teaching modules on mindfulness, narrative and reflective pedagogies, and cultural equity and inclusion. In 2012, she coedited a special issue of the *Archives of Psychiatric*

Nursing, applying the QSEN competencies to mental health nursing education. She continues to influence the scholarship and teaching-learning mindset of nurse educators around the world through her scholarly publications; international, national, and regional presentations; leadership in Caring Science; and service to the profession. Horton-Deutsch currently serves as a leadership mentor in the Nurse Faculty Leadership Academy through Sigma Theta Tau International.

Jan Anderson, EdD, MSN, RN, AHN-BC, Caritas Coach, is a faculty associate for the Watson Caring Science Institute and Director of the Caritas Coach Education Program. Anderson was formerly an adjunct professor and the Coordinator of the Watson Caring Science Center at the University of Colorado School of Nursing, and Director of the Santa Barbara City College Associate Degree Nursing Program, where she was also a professor. Anderson has both directed and taught the Caritas Coach Education Program (CCEP) for several years. A member of the first CCEP graduating class, Anderson has helped to develop and sustain the program, first with the Watson Caring Science Institute and then with the University of Colorado. The CCEP was the first program of its kind to be certified by the American Nurses Credentialing Center (ANCC) as an accredited Nursing Skills Competency Program (NSCP), in 2012.

Anderson has served on several boards, including Adventures in Caring, a local organization that helps to teach compassion in nursing; the Daughters of Charity, whose mission is to provide housing, education, and care for single women with children and seniors living in poverty in Santa Barbara; and the International Association for Human Caring as education chair. In her position as Director of the Associate Degree Nursing (ADN) Program at Santa Barbara City College in California, Anderson had the opportunity to work with faculty, staff, and students to integrate Dr. Watson's human caring theory and philosophy, as well as Caring Science, into all aspects of the nursing program. Anderson has also completed the International Certificate Program in Caring and Healing from the University of

Colorado Health Sciences Center School of Nursing; a 9-month telecourse for inter-spiritual mentors called "Deepening into Inter-spirituality" with Dr. Janet Quinn; and the Caritas HeartMath Literacy and HeartMath Coaching courses. Finally, Anderson completed the American Holistic Nurse's Association's certification for holistic nursing and the Nova Southeastern University's Fischler School of Education and Human Services' doctor of education program with an emphasis in nursing education. Anderson's dissertation examined the lived experience of the Caritas Coach.

CONTRIBUTING AUTHORS

Stephanie W. Ahmed, DNP, FNP-BC, DPNAP, Caritas Coach, serves as Director of Ambulatory Nursing at Brigham and Women's Hospital in Boston, Massachusetts. She is a family nurse practitioner with experience in areas ranging from community-based settings to surgical care. Ahmed is President of the Massachusetts Coalition of Nurse Practitioners and was inducted into the National Academies of Science as a distinguished fellow. She was Editor and contributing author for *DNP Education, Practice, and Policy: Redesigning Advanced Practice Roles for the 21st Century* (Springer Publishing Co., 2012). A member of the 2014 CCEP cohort, Ahmed believes that caritas is the antidote for the effects of health reform, humanizing the healthcare system and offering clinicians a framework to promote joy and resilience in practice.

Kino Xandro Anuddin, BSN, RN, CNN, HNB-B, Caritas Coach, currently serves as the Renal Nurse Educator at St. John Hospital and Medical Center in Detroit, Michigan. His role primarily involves providing and promoting health education for patients with renal disease, and facilitating training and competency among the nursing staff. Anuddin received his BSN degree from Ateneo de Zamboanga University in the Philippines and is board-certified in both nephrology and holistic nursing. Anuddin completed the CCEP through the Watson Caring Science Institute in April 2016.

Mark D. Beck, DNP, MSN, BS, RN-BC, CENP, certified Heart-Math trainer, WCSI postdoctoral fellow, Caritas Coach, has held leadership posts in nursing for more than three decades. He is currently an Assistant Professor at a Bay Area university, where, in addition to teaching, he is charged with designing an RN-to-BSN program with Caring Science as its framework. His prior position was Director of Clinical Education, Practice, and Informatics for a large integrated health system in Northern California. Beck has a background in adult and pediatric critical care, leadership development, and executive nursing practice, and is board-certified in nursing professional development as well as nurse executive practice. He is a certified HeartMath trainer and holds a Caritas Coach certificate from the Watson Caring Science Institute. He is currently a postdoctoral fellow at the Watson Caring Science Institute.

Katherine E. Belategui, BSN, RN, Caritas Coach, earned her BSN from Simmons College and began work as a staff nurse at Brigham and Women's Hospital in Boston, Massachusetts. She is passionate about caring for the hospital's neuroscience patient population and currently serves as a nurse in charge on the neuroscience intermediate care unit. She is an active member of the American Association of Neuroscience Nurses and Sigma Theta Tau International Honor Society. Belategui was a 2014–2015 Boston College Neuroscience Haley Scholar and is currently pursuing her MSN at the University of Massachusetts Boston. She earned her Caritas Coach certification in 2016 and is the Cochair of her unit's Caring Science Committee, designed to engage nurses in the principles and practice of Caring Science.

Christine Buckley, DNP, MBA, BSN, RN, CPHQ, NEA-BC, Caritas Coach, is Associate Chief Nursing Officer, Women's & Children's Services at UMass Memorial Medical Center—Memorial Campus in Worcester, Massachusetts. Buckley's nursing career spans more than 35 years in leadership, pediatrics, and critical care. She received her BSN in nursing from Boston College, her DNP from Massachusetts General Hospital Institute for Healthcare Professionals, and is a graduate of the executive MBA program at Boston University. She is board-certified as Nurse Executive-Advanced (NEA-BC), has achieved recognition as a Certified Professional in Healthcare Quality (CPHQ), and is a certified Caritas Coach. Buckley is a member of the Organization of Nurse Leaders and the American Organization of Nurse Executives.

Reid Byrne, MSN, MA, CNM, Caritas Coach, Reiki Master, CMT, is a Certified Nurse Midwife. After a career as a Communication Information Systems Officer in the United States Marine Corps, she earned an MA degree in practical theology from Colgate

Rochester Crozer Divinity School. She is a certified massage thera-pist and Reiki master. Byrne has guided many mothers and families through the powerful and transformative experience of pregnancy and childbirth in varied roles as a doula, homebirth apprentice midwife, obstetrical nurse, and soon as a certified nurse-midwife. She is the Public Relations and Marketing Chair in the Virginia affiliate of the American College of Nurse Midwives and is actively involved in local and statewide birth communities to support collaboration between birth professionals at all levels of care. Reid lives in Richmond, Virgin-ia, with her amazingly supportive husband and two beautiful children.

Jill Garabed-Hruska, BSCN, CAE, Caritas Coach, is a nursing instructor at Assiniboine Community College in Brandon, Manitoba. She has worked to incorporate holistic nursing practices throughout her nursing career. These have elevated clinical interactions with clients and their families. In 2016, Garabed-Hruska completed a 6-month Caritas Coach program through the University of Colorado based on the foundation of Jean Watson's Caring Science. Garabed-Hruska now weaves caring curriculum into the college's current practices. Garabed-Hruska's personal philosophy is that every interaction with any human being should leave the individual feeling valued. To maintain a healthy work-life balance, Garabed-Hruska enjoys traveling, cooking, and writing about reflective metaphors and how they apply to our lives. She also is passionate about collecting rocks and about spending time with her husband, grown daughters, grandson, and delightful dog—preferably outdoors while embracing the beauty of nature.

Joseph Giovannoni, DNP, APRN, WCSI postdoctoral scholar, Caritas Coach, is a Doctor of Nursing Practice at Joseph Giovannoni Inc. and a Watson Caring Science Institute postdoctoral scholar. Giovannoni is an advanced practice nurse with prescriptive author-ity, an AASECT board-certified sex therapist, and a clinical member of Association for the Treatment of Sexual Abusers. He provides holistic, compassionate, evidence-informed, patient-centered mental health treatment. He has integrated Watson's theory of Caring Sci-ence into his forensic practice. For the past 35 years he has conducted sex offense–specific evaluations and sex-offender cognitive behav-ioral groups under contracts with the State of Hawaii Judiciary. His practice consists of individual, couples, and family psychotherapy, and psycho-pharmacological management for mental disorders. He has lectured internationally and conducts Caring Science self-care workshops for healthcare science professionals, law-enforcement officers, forensic professionals, and others to help lower stress, prevent burnout, and sustain a healthy quality of life.

Lisa Goldberg, PhD, RN, Caritas Coach, is an Associate Professor at the School of Nursing Faculty of Health Professions, Dalhousie University. Her research and educational scholarship build on her expertise as a perinatal nurse with a disciplinary background in philosophy. Pragmatically and theoretically, nursing and philosophy align to drive innovative methodologies in feminist and queer phenomenology. Collectively, they provide tools for Goldberg to examine the practices of nurses in relation to women in the context of birth—specifically against the backdrop of power, gender, and heteronormativity. In 2014, upon completing the CCEP, Goldberg's scholarship broadened to examine the invisibility of LGBTQ+ identities in nursing through application of a Caring Science philosophy. This returns nursing to its foundational beginnings, inclusive of the compassion, reflexivity, and politicization so beautifully embodied in the works of Florence Nightingale.

Christine Griffin, MS, RN, CPN, master HearthMath trainer, Caritas Coach, is a Clinical Practice Specialist at Children's Hospital Colorado. From the role of bedside nurse to that of educator, Griffin has grasped the need for all care providers to build their nursing foundation in theory-based practice. She also understands on a very personal level the unique stressors that healthcare providers face and the need to build a practice of self-care and resiliency. Griffin became a Caritas Coach in 2010 and a HeartMath trainer 2 years later. Uniting an understanding of why we care for others with tools to manage stress has helped build and sustain the caring practices for Griffin, and subsequently others. Through all her experiences it has become crystal clear to Griffin that caregivers must take care of themselves first before managing the complexities of caring for others.

Heidi J. Hagle, RN, HN-BC, Caritas Coach, is a nurse at St. John Hospital and Medical Center. She started her career in nursing in 2001 working as a medical/surgical neurology/urology nurse. She was Assistant Clinical Manager for 3 years before she chose to step out of management, instead joining a preoperative/post anesthesia care unit, where she has been for 12 years. Hagle is a board-certified holistic nurse and a Caritas Coach. Being a Caritas Coach has helped her share her passion for Caring Science with everyone she encounters. Hagle has initiated music therapy into the perioperative patient experience and plans to continue expanding caring practices throughout the hospital. Currently she is working on her BSN and plans to continue her education further. Being a mother to three beautiful children is the most important part of her life.

Rachel Johnson-Koenke, LCSW, is a Research Social Worker and Caritas Coach at the Eastern Colorado Health Care System Department of Veterans Affairs and a doctoral student at the University of Colorado College of Nursing. Johnson-Koenke has practiced as a clinical social worker in healthcare systems for the past 9 years and as a research social worker for the past 5. She has been studying the role of social workers in chronic illness management and developing social work interventions to improve symptom burden and quality of life. She is interested in ways to bring Caring Science to social work practice and interdisciplinary teams. She lives in Denver with her husband, Chris, and daughter, Luna.

Lacey Lefere, MSN, BA, RN, AHN-BC, C-EFM, Caritas Coach, graduated from Central College in Pella, Iowa, in 2008 with a bachelor's degree. She pursued a career outside healthcare for a short time, but soon found nursing. She earned her MSN in 2012 from DePaul University in Chicago, Illinois. Lefere started as a floor nurse on an inpatient obstetrical unit in the Chicago area before moving to Detroit, Michigan and joining St. John Hospital & Medical Center, part of Ascension Health. There she has worked as a floor nurse and clinical nurse specialist, and now serves as the site's Magnet Program Director. Through inspirational mentors and working at an institution grounded in the theory of Caring Science as a Jean

Watson Caring Science affiliate, Lefere has developed a growing passion for holistic nursing and its essential future in healthcare. In her spare time, Lefere enjoys photography, reading, being outdoors, and spending time with her family.

Nancy Mathews, MS, BS, HeartMath trainer, Caritas Coach, is the Associate Director of the Watson Caring Science Center at the University of Colorado College of Nursing, assisting the endowed chair on strategic, operational, and outreach endeavors. She earned her undergraduate degree in sociology from the University of Wisconsin-Madison and her MS in computer information systems from the University of Wisconsin-Whitewater. She holds certifications as a Caritas Coach and HeartMath trainer. Mathews has an extensive background in international collaborations, relationship management, conference and event management, marketing, and program development. Through her leadership and her innovative spirit, she provides a vision for developing new partnerships and a resource for building strong relationships. Mathews revels in teaching and oversees the development of online courses in Caring Science, including the CCEP, which gives clinicians, educators, caregivers, and leaders the knowledge, experience, and informed practices of Caring Science and the theory of human caring.

Kathleen S. Oman, PhD, RN, FAEN, FAAN, Caritas Coach, is Professor and Chair of Pediatric Nursing at the University of Colorado College of Nursing and Children's Hospital Colorado. A life-long learner, Oman's professional expertise includes evidence-based practice, emergency nursing, ethics, and Caring Science. She teaches in the Caring Science track at the University of Colorado College of Nursing PhD program. At Children's Hospital Colorado, she supports the evidence-based practice program and assists with developing the caritas practice program. In her personal life, Oman enjoys hiking, golf, reading, and cooking. She has a great husband and a new puppy. She enjoys her work and her friends, and is grateful for all she has.

Nicholas J. Peterson, MSN, BSN, BA, RN, Caritas Coach, is an Ambulatory Nurse Educator at Brigham and Women's Hospital.

Peterson completed the CCEP in the spring of 2017. This experience was transformative both at work and in his home life. Peterson is an enthusiastic participant in the caritas initiative within the hospital community and is thrilled to share his experiences.

Diane Poulios, MA, RN, CHCR, AHN-BC, Caritas Coach, is a Nursing Recruitment Manager at Monmouth Medical Center, an affiliate of RWJBarnabas Health. Poulios earned her nursing degree at Georgetown University and started her career as an oncology nurse at Sloan Kettering Cancer Center in New York City. To complement conventional care and offer more of herself to her patients, Poulios learned various holistic modalities to alleviate their pain, anxiety, and fatigue. She became an oncology nurse educator after receiving her MA from NYU. She has published chapters, contributed to journals, presented at conferences, and lectured on cancer prevention, self-care, and holistic nursing. She has received multiple awards and was nominated for a New Jersey Governor's Award. Poulios became a nurse recruiter in 2000 to lead change and to champion the profession during a time of healthcare upheaval. Her belief in the nurse's role as the healing environment for the patient propels her recruitment and retention initiatives. Poulios attained her advanced holistic certification and recently became a certified health coach to demonstrate that healing starts with self.

Jennifer Reese, MD, Caritas Coach, is Associate Professor of Clinical Pediatrics in the section of pediatric hospital medicine at the University of Colorado School of Medicine. She is also the Interim Section Head and Medical Director of the section of pediatric hospital medicine and serves as the Inpatient Medical Director for Children's Hospital Colorado. On the clinical side she works as a pediatric hospitalist. Her administrative duties include quality and process improvement and clinical leadership, as well as developing and promoting programs that support wellness and resilience for healthcare providers. In 2015, Reese formed and now directs the University of Colorado School of Medicine Resilience Program for faculty, residents, and fellows. She completed her undergraduate degree and medical school at University of Washington in Seattle,

Washington, and her pediatric internship and residency at the University of Colorado School of Medicine and Children's Hospital Colorado. Since finishing residency, Reese has worked at Children's Hospital Colorado. Her passions include being a mother to her two sons, running, cycling, golfing, cooking, and traveling with her partner, David.

William Rosa, MS, RN, LMT, AHN-BC, AGPCNP-BC, CCRN-CMC, Caritas Coach, is a palliative care nurse practitioner Fellow at Memorial Sloan-Kettering Cancer Center in New York. He will begin his PhD studies at the University of Pennsylvania as a Robert Wood Johnson Future of Nursing scholar in the fall of 2017. He graduated magna cum laude with his BSN from the NYU Rory Meyers College of Nursing (2009) and as valedictorian of his MSN program at Hunter College (2014). Rosa is the Editor of two books on leadership and global health and author of more than 130 book chapters, journal and newspaper articles, and social media publications. He has been acknowledged with numerous honors, most recently as a national Rising Star in Nursing by *Modern Healthcare* (2017) and as a top-five finalist in the America's Most Amazing Nurse contest sponsored by *The Doctors* TV show and *Prevention* magazine. He has served multiple leadership roles for professional organizations and worked internationally with the Rwanda Human Resources for Health Program. Rosa is a Fellow of the New York Academy of Medicine.

TABLE OF CONTENTS

FOREWORD

"Every hospital should have an expert in human
caring on every unit."
–Binx Selby

How do you have an expert in human caring on every unit?

How do you cultivate a Caring Consciousness Culture in healthcare? A Caritas Consciousness (Love and Caring)?

How do you set your intentions to be authentically, mindfully, present in a given moment?

How do you experience a transpersonal caring moment?

How do you learn authentic heart-centered listening?

How do you cultivate practice of Loving Kindness, Compassion, and Equanimity for self/other? Our life? For your personal/professional circumstances? Our world? Our Planet?

How do you/we create and enter a new space, a new awakening, a new horizon for self/life purpose and service?

These rhetorical questions for our time invite us into territory that is existential, spiritual, metaphysical, sacred, and even mysterious. How do we find ways to live in "right-relation" with universal Source as ultimate healing, health, and wholeness for humanity? Over the past two decades, the discipline of nursing, which now informs other health-healing professions, has acknowledged that wholeness and human caring-healing cannot be fully addressed until theory, scholarship, and practice are situated within the evolved unitary-transformative paradigm (Koithan, Kreitzer, & Watson, 2017; Newman, Sime, & Corcoran-Perry, 1991; Phillips, 2017; Watson & Smith, 2002).

These unitary, sacred philosophical-ethical principles are transpersonal. The Caritas Coach program curriculum, which is congruent with Unitary Caring Science and Phillips' tenets (2017) of new theoretical unitary science, includes:

- Humans "*Belong*" to the infinite field of Universal Love— Drawing upon Levinas' Ethic of "Belonging" (Belonging comes before our separate Being; Levinas, 1969).

- The human spirit is infinite.

- Consciousness is nonlocal, beyond the physical brain.

- Consciousness transcends time, space, and physicality and goes beyond the moment, becoming part of the complex energetic pattern of one's life.

- Transpersonal caring moment is affected by one's consciousness, authenticity, energetic presence, and intentionality in a given moment.

- Transpersonal caring goes beyond itself and becomes part of the infinite, complex life pattern.

- Transpersonal caring moment can be a turning point for healing.

- Professional Caring Practices draw upon Energetic Caring Healing Modalities

(Koithan et al., 2017; Watson, 1999, 2005, 2008, 2012, 2017, 2018).

Horton-Deutsch and Anderson have collated the foundation for the Caritas Coach Educational Program, inviting readers into informed moral praxis. This program is grounded in the most mature disciplinary foundation to engage in compassionate caring-healing as a gift of self for Caritas leadership service for our life-world.

This time of turmoil and tumultuous upheaval in healthcare is an occasion for a major cosmic shift of consciousness for human caring, healing, and whole person/whole system shifts. Each of us is called forth to help birth and bring forth a new era for humanity that expands, elevates, and transcends the current, often noncaring, nonhumane practices in our challenging, changing world. As we awaken to a sustainable world future for humanity and Mother

Earth, we search for a way forward to make a difference, whether large or small.

Caritas Coaching and the vignettes here offer another way forward as a purposive invitation and inspiration for personal and professional transformation from within. In both small and grand ways, Caritas Coaches are making a difference. Why? Because the program provides an educational and cultural template for leadership and deep inner transformation for self-caring, compassion, loving-kindness, and equanimity for all. This deep philosophical foundation is translated into informed moral actions, concretely and energetically in situations and systems. Thus, the Caritas Coach projects and processes capture exemplary personal and professional accomplishments, which serve as a hopeful paradigm of possibility for humankind.

Individually and collectively, the Caritas Coach program and Coach exemplary accomplishments build upon the 10-year evolution and transformative success of this Watson Caring Science Institute (WCSI) program, which builds upon Unitary Caring Science and Theory and Philosophy of Transpersonal Caring. These Caritas Coach vignettes from leading educators, practitioners, and scholar-leaders reveal their inner-outer journey, resulting in deep change from within. The result is transformative, even revolutionary, toward constructive, nonconforming ways of Being/Doing/Knowing/ Becoming—Living Caritas—as the artistry of deepening, sustaining, and living-caring, healing, dignity, integrity, wholeness, for our shared humanity in harmony with Mother Earth.

What informs this Caritas Coach Program and Projects?

Caritas Coaches and the WCSI Coaching program build upon and expand timeless values, philosophy, theory, and ethic of caring-healing and Love, which touch the life force and human core of each coach and their inner/outer journey. The Caritas Coach program prepares Caritas leaders who both experientially and intellectually are equipped with a new language and who are able to give voice and informed moral praxis in their daily life-world—leading to a unitary caring consciousness of Diversity and Oneness, honoring the Sacred Circle of Life -Death.

Drs. Horton-Deutsch and Anderson have authored and edited an important record for this work, which calls upon Caritas Coaches and their personal/professional journey into a new worldview for humankind. It is through this Caritas Coaching and other related programs that, indeed, now and in the future: *"Every hospital can have an expert in human caring on every unit."*

–Jean Watson, PhD, RN, AHN-BC, FAAN, LL (AAN)

REFERENCES

Koithan, M., Kreitzer, M. J., & Watson, J. (2017). Linking the unitary paradigm to policy through a synthesis of caring science and integrative nursing. *NSQ, 30(3)*, 262–268.

Levinas, E. (1969). *Totality and infinity.* Pittsburgh, PA: Duquesne University.

Newman, M., Sime, A., & Corcoran-Perry, S. (1991). The focus of the discipline of nursing. *Advances in Nursing Science, 14(1)*, 1–6.

Phillips, J. (2017). New Rogerian theoretical thinking about unitary science. *Nursing Science Quarterly, 30(3)*, 223–226.

Watson, J. (1999). *Postmodern nursing and beyond.* Edinburgh, Scotland: Churchill-Livingstone.

Watson, J. (2005). *Caring science as sacred science.* Philadelphia, PA: F. A. Davis.

Watson, J. (2008). *Nursing. The philosophy and science of caring.* Boulder, CO: University Press of Colorado.

Watson, J. (2012). *Human caring science: A theory of nursing* (2nd ed.). Burlington, MA: Jones & Bartlett Learning.

Watson, J. (2017). Global caritas literacy. In S. Lee, P. Palmieri, & J. Watson (Eds.), *Global caring literacy* (pp. 3–11). New York, NY: Springer.

Watson, J. (2018). *Unitary caring science: The philosophy and praxis of nursing.* Boulder, CO: University Press of Colorado.

Watson, J. (in press). Integrative nursing and caring science: Universals of human caring and healing. In M. J. Kreitzer & M. Koithan, *Integrative nursing* (2nd ed.). New York, NY: Oxford Press.

Watson, J., & Smith, M. (2002). Caring science and the science of unitary human beings: A trans-theoretical discourse for nursing knowledge development. *Journal of Advanced Nursing, 37(5)*, 452–461.

INTRODUCTION

–Sara Horton-Deutsch, PhD, RN, FAAN, ANEF, Caritas Coach
–Jan Anderson, EdD, MSN, RN, AHN-BC, Caritas Coach

Nurses have always been the source of heart and healing in the healthcare system. In recent years, these roles and responsibilities have expanded to other formal and informal caregivers.

Care providers of all kinds have little opportunity to make sense of their own experiences. Being ill-prepared for the heavy toll of the work, we often end up depleted. Over time, to cope with the myriad complexities in providing care, we develop habits and routines to ground us. However, many of us reach a point in our careers where we find ourselves at a crossroads, realizing we can either accept things the way they are, leave, or search for a different way.

In this book, nurses and other formal and informal caregivers—including those in medicine, social work, and education—share deeply intimate stories about how they found a different way: by integrating Caring Science into their practice. Caring Science reconsiders science from an ontological perspective. It provides a scientific and philosophical context from which to explore, describe, and research human healing phenomena as integral to our humanity. By integrating Caring Science into their practice, these nurses reconnected with and strengthened their ethics and values, expanded their consciousness, and found new ways of being, becoming, knowing, and doing in all aspects of life.

The idea for this book emerged from an appreciative moment in the Caritas Coach Education Program (CCEP). (*Caritas*, from the Latin word meaning *to cherish*, means to care with love—with compassion, generosity, and spirit.) CCEP is a unique 6-month educational program based on the moral, ethical, philosophical, and practice principles of Caring Science. The program—launched in 2008 by Dr. Jean Watson and now overseen by Jan Anderson—is semi-structured, experiential, aesthetic, personal, ethical, and intellectual in nature. During a CCEP workshop in 2015, participants began sharing stories of their personal and professional transformations through Caring Science. These stories were so profound it seemed they should be shared more widely. And so this book was born. The authors and contributors hope this book will reawaken readers to the grace and beauty of a caring moment and the path to transpersonal caring, remind readers why they became caregivers in the first place, and help them reconnect with their purpose.

The first part of the book is an overview of the theory of human caring and Caring Science, a description of the CCEP, the CCEP curriculum, Caritas Coaching, and caritas ontological literacy, including the concepts of self-awareness, self-exploration, transpersonal care, reflective practice, and caring literacy.

The next five parts of the book, which share contributor stories, were sorted by focus. (Note that this is a fluid organization, as many of these stories transcend any particular characterization.) The categories are as follows:

- Caritas education in academic settings
- Caritas education in clinical settings
- Caritas praxis
- Caritas leadership (creating a foundation for praxis)
- Caritas leadership (creating a vision for the future)

All contributing authors were asked to contemplate and integrate responses to the following questions:

- What does it mean to become and be a Caritas Coach?
- How does Caring Science inform my thinking and practice?
- How do I manifest transpersonal caring in my practice? (Transpersonal caring is a higher form of "spiritual" caring created through caring moments.)
- How can I use caring literacy as a guide for my own professional development?
- How do self-awareness and reflection guide and sustain me?

The final part of the book provides a brief synthesis of the narratives and a path for moving forward in two ways:

- By expanding the ways knowledge becomes apparent (empirical, personal, aesthetic, and ethical) and thus deepening understanding
- By moving this deeper understanding into morally informed action

As these stories attest, transformations can be uncomfortable. But temporary discomfort is a small price to pay for reconnecting with one's health, wholeness, and humanity. In these stories, contributing authors share how they have learned and grown (and continue to learn and grow) through a lifelong spirit-filled journey. The stories explore how, through the study and practice of Caring Science, the contributing authors found new ways of relating to themselves and others, whether in teaching, research, education, or practice. They reveal how to break from habits and routine, find new meaning and purpose, and recall what draws us to the career in the first place. Finally, their stories illuminate what Dr. Jean Watson has espoused for many years:

> ...the practitioners of caring and healing require more personal work than ever before: because we practice who we are; we research who we are; we teach who we are; we live who we are. So, our very Being-Becoming more human and humane is what is at stake in healing work. (2005, p. 115)

Our lives have been transformed because we have embraced Caring Science as the foundation for our being, becoming, knowing, and doing in the world. We hope readers will be inspired by the stories of personal and professional transformation through the embodiment of Caring Science, and that they will be encouraged to seek their own inner and outer journey to health, healing, and wholeness.

REFERENCE

Watson, J. (2005). *Caring science as sacred science*. Philadelphia, PA: F. A. Davis Co.

Bringing the Philosophy, Ethic, and Practice of Caring Science Back into Healthcare

Caritas Coaching: An Overview

–Jan Anderson, EdD, MSN, RN, AHN-BC,
Caritas Coach

M any patients and families report feeling treated like a diagnosis or body system, or being spoken *at* (rather than spoken *with*) as their provider transcribes into a computer. At the same time, many nurses and other healthcare professionals report questioning why they went into healthcare when they lack the time to genuinely care for their patients.

Whether it's because we are in a rush to assess, intervene, diagnose, or prescribe, somewhere along the way, healthcare professionals have lost sight of the essence of their practice: caring. Caring is an essential aspect of the discipline of nursing and other healthcare professions. Caring nurtures the whole person and his or her environment, and is essential to the health and well-being of healthcare providers and those they care for. The goal of this book is to provide a path for bringing *caring* back into healthcare.

This book emphasizes *transpersonal caring*—a way of being fully with another person while staying mindful of *how* we are caring for them. Transpersonal caring reflects the fact that we are all connected and that what affects one of us also affects the other. It emphasizes the need to balance medical science with Caring Science. It is about bringing humanity back into healthcare by emphasizing the health, healing, and wholeness of the person, family, and community.

The chapters in this book explore each author's individual journey toward discovering and practicing transpersonal caring. To provide readers with a foundation for understanding these stories, this chapter covers:

- An overview of the theory of human caring and Caring Science
- An explanation of the Caritas Coach Education Program (CCEP) and the principles and practices that guide it
- Caring literacies—the human attributes necessary to provide care based in consciousness, intention, and love for self and other (*other* refers to any human being—e.g., patients, families, visitors, coworkers, volunteers, etc.).

THE THEORY OF HUMAN CARING

The theory of human caring was developed by Dr. Jean Watson in the mid-1970s. She recognized the need for a theoretical foundation and disciplinary framework that more explicitly described the bio-genic (life-giving and life-receiving) (Halldorsdottir, 1991) qualities of caring and healing as they applied to the discipline of nursing. Watson first published her theory in 1979 in *Nursing: The Philosophy and Science of Caring*.

Caring Science is as much about the practitioner as it is about the practice—transforming from a mechanistic, objective, and empirically based practice to a more holistic, human, compassionate approach (Watson, 1999a, 2008). The theory is based on the premise that the nurse's mission is to care for and to heal self and humanity. A humanistic practice requires human-to-human connections and interactions that emphasize the importance, value, and dignity of each unique and precious human, with the goal of healing rather than solely treating and curing (Watson, 2008). The theory provides a unique vision for nurses and all healthcare providers that complements the dominant medical model. This balance of the art and science of nursing provides the discipline of nursing with a renewed vision of purpose and practice.

Caring Science: Healthcare as a Sacred Act

Watson's life work has been to expand and clarify her original theory into one that is more inclusive and meaningful to all healthcare professionals, renaming the theory of human caring to *Caring Science*. Caring Science is based in the same premises and principles as the theory of human caring but also includes "new understandings of science, forms of inquiry, methods and practices, reigniting connections between science, art, spirituality, and restoring values, ethics and new relationships between heart sciences, and humanities and the arts for healing purposes" (Medscape, 2005, p. 1). Healing does not refer solely to a physical cure; rather, it is described from the transpersonal perspective as the "preservation of humanity and wholeness" (Watson, 1999b, p. 118). Healing occurs in relationship with oneself and

another, and as alignment—being in harmony internally and exter-
nally, and at-one-ment with *source*. Watson (2008) defines *source* as
"access to a deeper/higher energy source, i.e. one's God." She notes
that this "is as important to healing as are our conventional treatment approaches, and is possibly even more powerful in the long-
run" (1999b, p. 115), emphasizing a sacred dimension of care.

Healthcare practice that includes these healing goals are now defined by the concept of *caritas*—an integration of love and care that
reminds us of the sacred work of healthcare and is manifested as
caritas consciousness. Humanism and caritas shift healthcare from
a task orientation to a focus on the importance of the subjective
inner life of human beings as embodied spirits. This further emphasizes the underlying spiritual and sacred aspects of caregivers, their
practice, and those in their care. In this way, healthcare is viewed as
an "ethical covenant" (Watson, 2008, p. 2) with the community and
the world, and healthcare practice becomes a series of sacred acts
that touch the human soul as well as the physical body.

TRANSPERSONAL RELATIONSHIPS

The subjective inner life of each of us forms the basis for the development of deep personal connections. These define transpersonal
relationships and serve as sources for health and healing. Transpersonal relationships are relationships built on mutual trust, respect,
and honor. *Transpersonal* means each person is equal, recognized,
respected, and honored for his or her contribution, wholeness, and
special gifts and talents. The caring transpersonal relationship results
in a biogenic (life-giving) experience. In contrast, the noncaring
relationship results in a *biocidic* (life-destroying) experience. Noncaring as described by Swanson (1999) results in humiliation, fear,
a sense of loss of control, desperation, helplessness, alienation, and
vulnerability. These biocidic experiences are life-destroying for all
involved, including healthcare practitioners and those they care for.

Noncaring also represents caritas illiteracy and is an ethical failure for the profession (Watson, 2008).

As we begin to more fully understand and recognize the effects of caring and noncaring on all those involved, we begin to realize that Caring Science becomes an ontology, or way of being and becoming, knowing, and doing. We also begin to see that caritas ontological literacy (Lee, Palmieri, & Watson, 2017) becomes an ethical and moral imperative for all healthcare professions.

Being and becoming means being and becoming more human and humane; *doing* becomes a way of taking action based on thoughtful biogenic decisions and mindful, authentic, and loving communication and presence (Watson, 2008); and *knowing* represents the many ways we learn about what we see, hear, feel, and experience through the lens of Caring Science. The caritas practitioner walks alongside the other, assisting as needed and empowering all to evolve toward more wholeness, a higher consciousness, and optimum health.

To see, understand, and develop transpersonal relationships, healthcare providers expand their focus from strictly empirical ways of knowing to multiple ways of knowing, including:

- Ethical
- Aesthetic
- Personal
- Experiential
- Intuitive
- Sociopolitical (Zander, 2007)
- Unknowing (approaching complex realities of people and their worldview from a "position of openness" [Munhall, 1993, p. 125])

These many ways of knowing self and other acknowledge that all individuals come with life histories and experiences that affect health, well-being, and healing, shifting the focus of healthcare practice toward learning from, and connecting with, the self and other. This creates deeper and more meaningful connections extending from self to other to the community and beyond.

The caritas practitioner's relationship with self is the first step in the lifelong search for evolved consciousness, harmony, and alignment. Self-care is based on reflective caring-healing practices to promote and sustain the development of self-awareness, mindfulness, and caritas consciousness. Reflective practices help each person to love and accept the self and to also be willing to take the necessary steps to transform for the better—a repatterning toward health and healing.

In this way, each person becomes his or her optimal self by:

- Living with caritas consciousness and intentionality

- Knowing that we are all part of humanity and have something to contribute

- Realigning each of us to the human condition and to our shared struggles, hopes, and dreams

- Sustaining a lifelong journey towards health, healing, wholeness, and compassion

As we accept and treat ourselves with loving-kindness, equanimity, and compassion, we are able to do the same for the other. As we surrender to what is, we are able to be present in the moment, to be grateful for the lessons each connection and interaction brings to us, and to live life more fully and joyfully. As a result, the caritas practitioner focuses on self and self-care and not on controlling or directing others. With self-care as a focus, the Caring Science practitioner more fully recognizes and embraces her or his humanness and the humanness of others, enabling each to be who they are: authentic, unique, and precious.

THE CARITAS COACH EDUCATION PROGRAM

The Watson Caring Science Institute (WCSI) is a nonprofit organization created by Dr. Jean Watson and a handful of Caring Science scholars and clinicians. The WCSI goal is to transform healthcare through Caring Science, promote Caring Science research, and nurture and support professional nursing. (For more information, see https://www.watsoncaringscience.org/.) The Caritas Coach Education Program (CCEP) was developed by WCSI in 2008 to address the need for an expanded nurse coach role. The program relies on Caring Science as the framework for teaching, learning, and modeling the theory. CCEP is accredited by the American Nurses Credentialing Center (ANCC) as a nursing skills competency program and has certified more than 350 Caritas Coaches nationally and internationally.

CCEP is 6-month educational program that uses the caritas model of advanced teaching and learning in caring curriculum. Advanced teaching and learning includes the transpersonal aspects of developing helping-trusting relationships, working from the other's frame of reference, and finding meaning. In this way, teaching and learning become more personalized, individualized, and respectful (Watson, 2008). Caring curriculum emphasizes the development of the students as a person first and healthcare professional second. Teaching and learning in CCEP are structured as a caritas journey that occurs through active student engagement. The goal of the Caring Science curriculum is to provide a foundation for caring practice and education by creating a professional practice based on the following (Hills & Watson, 2011; Watson, 2008):

- Internal dialogue
- Reflection
- Awareness
- Consciousness
- Health
- Care

This includes reading, reflection, experience, and faculty relationships. It also occurs through knowledge and wisdom beyond intellectual understanding through objectives and subjectives of learning and teaching. Subjectives address the deeper meaning and feeling of learning and teaching; they also relate to the idea of ontology—in other words, the idea that we learn and teach how to be and become, do, and know rather than focusing simply on the objectives or empirical understanding or cognition (Hills & Watson, 2011). Caring Science curriculum transforms teaching and learning from traditional classroom teaching methodology to encompass multiple ways of knowing, which are considered valid and important to the teaching/learning process, including such methodologies as art, music, imagery, poetry, and narrative learning. The integration of the objective and subjective experience in CCEP helps to develop caritas literacy to care for, heal, and touch both the human spirit and the physical body (MacNeil & Evans, 2005). Healthcare professionals working from a Caring Science perspective recognize that literacy involves more than mere skills; it is the ability to integrate knowledge, attitudes, and values as a way of living (Watson, 2008).

This caritas journey promotes learning, teaching, and self-healing through the loving and supportive network that is the caritas community. As relationships deepen and students become more open to learning, they remember what brought them into nursing and healthcare and redefine their practice and lives with Caring Science as the foundation. They find confidence and comfort through learning and connections made in the caritas community, and they discover they have a new voice for sharing what nurses and other healthcare professionals do that is crucial in health and healing. Their practice transforms as caritas literacy helps them find their higher calling—the spirituality of providing sacred care to those in need.

THE CARITAS COACH

The Caritas Coach program expands the current view of coaching to include a focus on the health and healing of the coach self as a necessary first step to coaching another. This unique form of coaching begins with the inner work needed to be more self-aware, self-knowledge-able, intentional, conscious, and well. This in turn requires love, compassion, and equanimity for self. Self-care is seen as a foundation for caring for and coaching another.

Self-care and self-growth occur in a circular process as opposed to a linear one. As the Caritas Coach cares for the self—learning to love and accept self—he or she evolves into a more loving, compassionate human being who is better able to guide others to do the same. Every connection and interaction reflects back to the Caritas Coach and the other as lessons to be learned and experienced.

The Caritas Coach coaches self and other through "advanced teaching/learning" (Watson, 2008, p. 31). This can occur only in a transpersonal relationship, working from the perspective of the ones being coached (the *coachees*), as they become aware of "self-iden-tified issues and needs and their own inner goals [and] self-defined [and] self-motivated pursuits" (Watson, 2008, p. 127). In this way, the Caritas Coach relationship is one of walking alongside—Watson calls it the "I-thou" relationship (Watson, 2008, p. 81)—with both the coach and the coachee learning and teaching through the sharing of heart, spirit, and experience.

These foundations of equality, respect, honor, and wholeness lead to deep connections on a "spirit-to-spirit level with another, beyond personality, physical appearance, disease, diagnosis, even presenting behavior" (Watson, 2008, p. 82). It is in these deep connections that the transpersonal moment is created: a sacred space that offers access to all healing, learning, and growth possibilities and potentials to affect each person in that moment (Watson, 2008). All relationships—personal, professional, communal, and global—represent opportunities to create transpersonal caring moments, positively affecting those involved and the larger environment and culture. In this way, the Caritas Coach promotes the transformation of health-care systems and beyond, from the inside out (Watson, 2008).

Caritas Coaching is a spiritual endeavor. It acknowledges and treasures the spirit and soul of each person and appreciates that healing is a transformation or evolution of consciousness or spirit toward biogenic energies. As we more fully integrate spirituality, love, and compassion into our lives, we gain confidence that the caritas philosophy provides answers to the deeper questions we often ask ourselves:

- Who am I?
- Why am I here?
- What is my purpose?
- How can I make a difference?
- What is health and healing?
- How do I effect care and healing for those in my care?
- How can I change this experience?
- And so on

To become a Caritas Coach means to become a lifelong learner of what it means to be more fully who we are through our humanness using the core concepts of Caring Science as our guide.

CARITAS ONTOLOGICAL LITERACY

Watson describes the caritas ontological literacies "as intentional, cultivated, and learned approaches(s) to the whole person" (2008, p. 281) to emphasize that these literacies can be taught and learned. This description also helps us to distinguish the human attributes necessary to provide care based in Caring Science. Heart-centered intelligence and the cultivation of caritas consciousness move each of us toward a recognition and appreciation of our own humanity and the humanity of another (Watson, 2008). The Caritas Coach Education Program vision is to promote and strengthen caritas literacy to provide care based in Caring Science.

Caritas does not solely define behavior; it describes our intentions, attitudes, ethics, and values. The 10 Caritas Processes (formerly known as 10 Carative Factors) provide the basis for caritas ontological literacy.

———————— 10 CARITAS PROCESSES ————————

1. Practicing loving-kindness and equanimity for self and other

2. Being authentically present; enabling/sustaining/honoring deep belief system and subjective world of self/other

3. Cultivating one's own spiritual practices; deepening self-awareness, going beyond "ego-self"

4. Developing and sustaining a helping-trusting, authentic caring relationship

5. Being present to, and supportive of, the expression of positive and negative feelings as a connection with deeper spirit of self and the one-being-cared-for

6. Creative use of self and all ways of knowing/being/doing as part of the caring process (engaging in artistry of caring-healing practices)

7. Engaging in genuine teaching-learning experiences within context of caring relationship—attend to whole person and subjective meaning; attempt to stay within other's frame of reference (evolve toward "coaching" role vs. conventional imparting of information)

8. Creating a healing environment at all levels (physical, nonphysical, subtle environment of energy and consciousness whereby wholeness, beauty, comfort, dignity, and peace are potentiated [Being/Becoming the environment])

9. Reverentially and respectfully assisting with basic needs; holding an intentional, caring consciousness of touching and working with the embodied spirit of another, honoring unity of Being; allowing for spirit-filled connection

10. Opening and attending to spiritual, mysterious, unknown existential dimensions of life-death-suffering; "allowing for a miracle"

(Watson, 2008)

These 10 processes are described as the core of nursing and healthcare (Watson, 2008). *Core* refers to those aspects of caring for self and other that do not change. For example, Caritas Process 1, "Practicing loving-kindness and equanimity for self and other" (Watson, 2008, p. 47), generates several caritas literacies, including "opens to connecting with self, others, environment, and universe; model's self-care and caring for others; acknowledges acts of kindness; treats others with kindness; honors own and other's gifts and talents..." (Watson, 2008, p. 282). These core caritas literacies remain constant, transcending time, space, place, and occasion.

In contrast, the *trim* of practicing caring for self and other does change. Trim describes the content that is traditionally taught in healthcare education: "knowledge, technology, skills and activities" (Sitzman & Watson, 2013, p. 34). For example, with the rapid growth and pace of technology, computers and electronic records have revolutionized healthcare. These would be considered the *trim* of healthcare. At the same time, these advances have changed how care is provided and received, shifting the focus away from each human—those caring and those being cared for—and toward technology.

In all interactions, caritas literacies, being fluent in Caring Science, always focus on connecting through presence, authenticity, consciousness, loving-kindness, respectful communication, and so on. These literacies connect the science with the art of caring for self and other and are based in self-care, self-awareness, self-growth, and an openness of spirit.

Both the core and the trim are important to providing healthcare that is up to date and focused on each human. Caritas literacy attends to the "heart and emotions" of caring for self and other. It reminds us that caring for the other is not just applying skills—diagnosing and treating. It is being more fully present with self and other, and providing a way of living based in health, wholeness, and humanness. This way of living reconnects us with our purpose and values more intentionally, and helps us to care for ourselves and each other.

Work in caritas ontological literacy continues to evolve. The most recent work by Lee, Palmieri, and Watson (2017) offers insights into caritas literacy from a global perspective by experts around the world. The original caritas literacy project, created by a subgroup of the International Caritas Consortium in June 2007, can provide some context for the growth and evolution of caring literacy. Anderson (2014) also explores the relationships between what she calls the Caritas Coach ontological literacies, as they relate to the Nurse Coach Practice Competencies and the ANA Standards for Nursing, to help us to further define what it means to be caring literate.

RELATING CARITAS COACH ONTOLOGICAL LITERACIES TO NURSE COACH PRACTICE COMPETENCIES AND ANA STANDARDS

Caritas Coach ontological literacies integrate and reflect the American Nurses Association's (ANA's) Standards of Nursing Practice and complement the Nurse Coach Practice Competencies (Dossey, Hess, Southard, Luck, Schaub, & Bark, 2013).

The ANA standards guide nursing practice. These standards are divided into two categories: Standards of Practice and Standards of Professional Performance. They revolve around nursing processes (assessment, diagnosis, outcomes identification, planning, implementation, and evaluations) and performance (ethics, education, evidence-based practice, research, and so on). The Nurse Coach Practice Competencies are aligned with the ANA Standards of Nursing Practice, with a focus on the role and competencies of the nurse coach.

Caritas literacy, however—while congruent with the aforementioned standards and competencies—begins with a focus on "self-healing, self-growth and deliberate spiritual practices" (Watson, 2008, pp. 22–23) and arises from the Caritas Processes, with the goal of striving to become more human, kind, loving, and compassionate in the world, thus promoting health and healing.

CARITAS COACH ONTOLOGICAL LITERACIES	NURSE COACH PRACTICE COMPETENCIES	ANA STANDARDS
Integration of Caritas Processes and Literacies: Connects with self and others Validates uniqueness of self and others Honors own and others' gifts and talents Recognizes vulnerabilities in self and others Treats self and others with loving-kindness Listens with respect and genuine concern for others Demonstrates respect for self and others Listens to others Honors the human dignity of self and others Demonstrates genuine interest in others Enters into the experience to explore possibilities in the moment and in the relationship	**Assessment** Presence Relationship Communication Learning and coaching readiness Use of resources	**ANA** **Standard 1** Assessment
Integration of Caritas Processes and Literacies: Practices willingness to explore own feelings, beliefs, and values for self-growth Practices discernment in evaluating circumstances and situations rather than being judgmental Holds others with unconditional love and regard Holds sacred space of healing for others in their time of need Engages in effective, loving communication that promotes healthy living Engages in proactive problem-solving Engages in activities that maximize independence and individual freedom Engages in activities that promote safe, ethical, mature, and healthy growth experiences	**Diagnosis** Clarifies, confirms, and tracks client issues, concerns, and opportunities	**ANA** **Standard 2** Diagnosis

CARITAS COACH ONTOLOGICAL LITERACIES	NURSE COACH PRACTICE COMPETENCIES	ANA STANDARDS
Integration of Caritas Processes and Literacies: Creates and holds a sacred space for unfolding and emerging Acknowledges healing as an inner journey Allows for uncertainty and the unknown Encourages narrative and storytelling as a way to express understanding Allows the story to emerge, change, and grow Encourages full expression of sensations, feelings, thoughts, ideas, emotions, beliefs, and values to explore understanding and meaning Encourages reflection on feelings and experiences Helps others see some good aspects of their situation Accepts and helps others deal with negative feelings Participates in collaborative co-creation Helps others understand how they are thinking about their illness and health Helps others formulate and give voice to questions and concerns	**Outcomes Identification** Formulates goals with client that lead to change	**ANA Standard 3** Outcomes Identification
Integration of Caritas Processes and Literacies: Creates and holds a sacred space for unfolding and emerging Acknowledges healing as an inner journey Allows for uncertainty and the unknown Encourages narrative and storytelling as a way to express understanding Allows the story to emerge, change, and grow Encourages full expression of sensations, feelings, thoughts, ideas, emotions, beliefs, and values to explore understanding and meaning Encourages reflection on feelings and experiences Helps others see some good aspects of their situation Accepts and helps others deal with their negative feelings Participates in collaborative co-creation Helps others understand how they are thinking about their illness and health Helps others formulate and give voice to questions and concerns	**Planning** Identifies strategies to meet goals with client Creates action plan with clearly defined steps and anticipated results Explores obstacles Adjusts plan with client	**ANA Standard 4** Planning

continues

CARITAS COACH ONTOLOGICAL LITERACIES	NURSE COACH PRACTICE COMPETENCIES	ANA STANDARDS
Integration of Caritas Processes and Literacies: Creates and holds a sacred space for unfolding and emerging Acknowledges healing as an inner journey Allows for uncertainty and the unknown Encourages narrative and storytelling as a way to express understanding Allows the story to emerge, change, and grow Encourages full expression of sensations, feelings, thoughts, ideas, emotions, beliefs, and values to explore understanding and meaning Encourages reflection on feelings and experiences Offers blessings, prayer, and spiritual expression as appropriate Helps others see some good aspects of their situation Actively listens and lets energy flow through self without becoming consumed by others' feelings Accepts and helps others deal with their negative feelings	**Implementation** Present Grounded Centered Reviews client status and progress Explores outcomes and challenges Supports client Acknowledges strengths for change Uses an open, interested, and reflective approach Uses silence and reflection Trusts intuition and client perceptions Draws upon energy field or system Creates safe, supportive environment Exhibits honesty, sincerity, and integrity Respects client Provides ongoing support Obtains consent Uses a variety of strategies Looks for meaning using deep listening, communication, and powerful questioning	**ANA Standard 5** Implementation

CARITAS COACH ONTOLOGICAL LITERACIES	NURSE COACH PRACTICE COMPETENCIES	ANA STANDARDS
Integration of Caritas Processes and Literacies: Acknowledges acts of kindness Honors own and others' gifts and talents Recognizes vulnerabilities in self and others Listens respectfully and with genuine concern to others Demonstrates respect for self and others Respects others Honors the human dignity of self and others Practices self-reflection Demonstrates willingness to explore own feelings, beliefs, and values for self-growth Practices self-reflection Holds others with unconditional love and regard Brings full, honest, and genuine self to relationships Demonstrates sensitivity and openness to others Creates and holds sacred space Encourages reflection of feelings and experiences Integrates aesthetic knowledge for full expression of caring arts and sciences Views others as an integrated whole Respects others' unique individual needs Respects others' perceptions of the world and need for privacy Nurtures and supports hope Shows respect for things that have meaning to others	**Evaluation** Evaluates strategies and outcomes Supports client autonomy Documents	**ANA Standard 6** Evaluation
Integration of Caritas Processes and Literacies: Acknowledges acts of kindness Honors own and others' gifts and talents Recognizes vulnerabilities in self and others Listens respectfully and with genuine concern to others Demonstrates respect for self and others Respects others Honors the human dignity of self and others Practices self-reflection Demonstrates willingness to explore own feelings, beliefs, and values for self-growth Practices self-reflection	**Ethics** Follows the ANA Code of Ethics Respects client's rights, autonomy, dignity, values, and beliefs Values all life experiences as opportunities to find personal meaning and cultivate self-awareness, self-reflection, and growth Maintains client confidentiality	**ANA Standard 7** Ethics

continues

CARITAS COACH ONTOLOGICAL LITERACIES	NURSE COACH PRACTICE COMPETENCIES	ANA STANDARDS
Holds others with unconditional love and regard Brings full, honest, and genuine self to relationships Demonstrates sensitivity and openness to others Creates and holds sacred space Encourages reflection of feelings and experiences Integrates aesthetic knowledge for full expression of caring arts and sciences Views others as an integrated whole Respects others' unique individual needs Respects others' perceptions of the world and need for privacy Nurtures and supports hope Shows respect for things that have meaning to others		
Integration of Caritas Processes and Literacies: Engages in genuine teaching-learning experiences that attend to unity of being and meaning Participates in collegial/collaborative co-creation Expands self-knowledge in ways that engage in the artistry of caring-healing practices Engages in practices and rituals to promote spiritual growth Develops meaningful rituals for practicing gratitude, forgiveness, surrender, and compassion Cultivates transpersonal self toward a more full consciousness and heart-centeredness	**Education** Participates in ongoing educational activities to enhance role Documents and maintains evidence of competence Develops knowledge base	**ANA** **Standard 8** Education
Integration of Caritas Processes and Literacies: Integrates aesthetic, ethical, empirical, personal, and metaphysical ways of knowing with creative, imaginative, and critical thinking for full expression of caring arts and sciences Interacts with caring arts and sciences to promote healing and wholeness	**Evidence-Based Practice and Research** Uses evidence to guide and enhance practice Participates in research	**ANA** **Standard 9** Evidence-Based Practice and Research
Integration of Caritas Processes and Literacies: Engages in communication that promotes healthy living Engages in effective, loving communication Engages in proactive problem-solving Engages in activities that maximize independence Engages in activities that promote safe, ethical, mature, healthy growth experiences Acknowledges healing as an inner journey	**Quality of Practice** Contributes to education of others Documents Uses creativity and innovation in practice Analyzes organizational barriers Advocates for nurse coaching	**ANA** **Standard 10** Quality of Practice

CARITAS COACH ONTOLOGICAL LITERACIES	NURSE COACH PRACTICE COMPETENCIES	ANA STANDARDS
Helps others explore alternate ways to find new meaning in their situations and life journeys in dealing with their health and self-healing approaches Helps others formulate and give voice to questions and concerns to ask healthcare professionals Nurtures and supports hope		
Integration of Caritas Processes and Literacies: Is able to read the field when entering into the life space or field of another Is able to be present with as well as do for others Accurately identifies and addresses person by name Maintains eye contact as appropriate for person and cultural meaning and sensitivity Accurately detects others' feelings Stays within others' frame of reference Invites and authentically listens to the inner meaning and subjective story of others Authentically listens and hears behind the words Holds others with an attitude of unconditional loving-kindness, equanimity, dignity, and regard Is able to be with silence, waiting for others to reflect before responding to questions and allowing others' inner thoughts to emerge Responds to others' feelings and moods verbally and nonverbally with authentic affective congruence	**Communication** Uses skillful communication	**ANA Standard 11** Communication
Integration of Caritas Processes and Literacies: Practices Caritas Coaching aimed toward accountability and compassionate service in personal life, clinical and caregiving practice, teaching settings, and leadership roles (in addition to the preceding caritas competencies and literacies)	**Leadership** Advances role of nurse coach Develops leadership skills in all ways Promotes success of others Displays a passion for nurse coaching Accepts mistakes made Defines a clear vision, goals, and plans, and progress toward all three	**ANA Standard 12** Leadership

continues

CARITAS COACH ONTOLOGICAL LITERACIES	NURSE COACH PRACTICE COMPETENCIES	ANA STANDARDS
Integration of Caritas Processes and Literacies:	**Collaboration**	**ANA**
Practices willingness to explores one's feelings, beliefs, and values for self-growth	Communicates effectively	**Standard 13**
Practices discernment in evaluating circumstances and situations rather than being judgmental	Works collaboratively	Collaboration
Holds others with unconditional love and regard		
Holds sacred space of healing for others in their time of need		
Engages in effective, loving communication that promotes healthy living		
Engages in proactive problem-solving		
Engages in activities that maximize independence and individual freedom		
Engages in activities that promote safe, ethical, mature, and healthy growth experiences		
Is able to read the field when entering into the life space or field of another		
Is able to be present; be with as well as do for others		
Accurately identifies and addresses person by name		
Maintains eye contact as appropriate for person and cultural meaning and sensitivity		
Accurately detects others' feelings		
Stays within others' frame of reference		
Invites and authentically listens to the inner meaning and subjective story of others		
Authentically listens and hears behind the words		
Holds others with an attitude of unconditional loving-kindness, equanimity, dignity, and regard		
Is able to be with silence, waiting for others to reflect before responding to questions and allowing others' inner thoughts to emerge		
Responds to others' feelings and moods verbally and nonverbally with authentic affective congruence		
Is able to read the field when entering into the life space or field of another		

CARITAS COACH ONTOLOGICAL LITERACIES	NURSE COACH PRACTICE COMPETENCIES	ANA STANDARDS
Integration of Caritas Processes and Literacies: Promotes the evolutionary Caritas Coaching journey that embraces transformative being/becoming Caritas Coaches in action through continued study, networking, and use of resources Expresses the caritas lived experience through aesthetic-experiential-intellectual forms that enhance the understanding of caring and loving-kindness underpinning Caritas Coaching practices Describes the concepts of the theory of human caring and Caring Science as a modality for improving conscious, intentional, and heart-centered caritas practices Assimilates the 10 Caritas Processes and Caring Science core concepts in personal and professional Caritas Coaching role Develops a working Caritas Coaching philosophy or framework based on the theory of human caring and Caring Science	**Professional Practice Evaluation** Uses nurse coach framework and publications for practice Is culturally and spiritually sensitive in all aspects of practice Evaluates self Pursues certification Advances practice with self-development Receives coaching Uses research for practice	**ANA Standard 14** Professional Practice Evaluation
Integration of Caritas Processes and Literacies: Follows professional nursing practice that is grounded in ethics Promotes the evolutionary Caritas Coaching journey that embraces transformative being/becoming Caritas Coaches in action through continued study, networking, and use of resources	**Resource Utilization** Practices with safety, effectiveness, availability, cost-awareness, benefits, efficiencies, and impact Assists clients with identifying and securing resources	**ANA Standard 15** Resource Utilization
Integration of Caritas Processes and Literacies: Creates space for human connections to occur Participates in caring-healing consciousness Creates caring intentions Creates a healing environment, attending to nurse as environment, others as unique person, light, art, water, noise, cleanliness, privacy, nutrition, beauty, safety, hand washing, comfort measures, others' time frames, and others' routines and rituals Is available Pays attention to others when they are talking Anticipates others' needs	**Environmental Health** Understands internal and external healthy environments Recognizes individual aspects to internal and external environments Considers self and client environment and effect on goal achievement	**ANA Standard 16** Environmental Health

The Nurse Coach Practice Competencies and Caritas Coaching share a holistic perspective with a focus on wellness and health promotion. Nurse coaching focuses on change. So too does Caritas Coaching—although change is viewed through the Caring Science lens—as an internal transformation or repatterning. This internal transformation promotes an alignment of thoughts, feelings, actions, and intentions, leading to an expanded consciousness, health, and wellness.

Caritas literacy can be described as a fluency of the human spirit, whereas competency focuses on proficiency with a skill or a task. Competency confines both process and content to a linear, sequenced process with a focus on problem-solving. In contrast, Caritas Coaching is a circular process that explores and deepens the human relationship and attends to the unknown potentials for those in relationship, with the ultimate aim of co-creation and solution-finding.

Caritas Coaching is a way of being, becoming, knowing, and doing that cannot be scripted or achieved by following specific steps or sequences. Additionally, Caritas Coaching is inclusive and occurs in all settings—not only with those in our care, but with ourselves, our coworkers, our loved ones, and others. It is not just a role that is fulfilled by registered nurses to coach patients. Caritas Coaching is a spiritual journey toward finding purpose, alignment in life, and an opportunity to make a difference.

FINAL REFLECTIONS

Caritas ontological literacy and caring-healing practices offer a way to approach life and healthcare practice with a more balanced, loving, and compassionate spirit, knowing that we can make a positive difference through deep connection, caritas consciousness, and healing.

A commitment and dedication to a lifelong caritas journey begins with the courage to take the necessary transformative path toward openness, authenticity, acceptance, presence, and wellness. Each chapter in this book represents such a journey toward caritas literacy. Contributing authors have shared their personal and professional successes and struggles, their insights into how to infuse Caring Science into life and healthcare practice, and the tremendous rewards and insights gained on their unique and life-changing journeys.

REFERENCES

Anderson, J. (2014). Unpublished dissertation: *Exploring application of the Caritas Coach role in nursing practice*. Abraham S. Fischler School of Education and Human Services, Nova Southeastern University.

Dossey, B. M., Hess, D. R., Southard, M. E., Luck, S., Schaub, B. G., & Bark, L. (2013). *The art & science of nursing coaching: The provider's guide to coaching scope and competencies*. Silver Spring, MD: American Nurses Association.

Halldorsdottir, S. (1991). Five basic modes of being with another. *National League of Nursing Publications, (15-2401)*, 37–49.

Hills, M., & Watson, J. (2011). *Creating a caring science curriculum: An emancipatory pedagogy for nursing*. New York, NY: Springer Publishing Co.

Lee, S., Palmieri, P., & Watson, J. (2017). *Global advances in human caring literacy*. New York, NY: Springer Publishing Co.

MacNeil, M. S., & Evans, M. (2005). The pedagogy of caring in nursing education. *International Journal for Human Caring, 9*(4), 45–51.

Medscape. (September 30, 2005). Caring science and the caritas field: Our path. Retrieved from https://www.medscape.com/viewarticle/513614

Munhall, P. L. (1993). Unknowing: Toward another pattern of knowing in nursing. *Nursing Outlook, 41*, 125–128.

Sitzman, K., & Watson, J. (2013). *Caring science, mindful practice: Implementing Watson's human caring theory*. New York, NY: Springer Publishing Co.

Swanson, K. (1999). What is known about caring in nursing research: A literary meta-analysis. In A. S. Hinshaw, S. L. Feetham, & J. L. F. Shaver (Eds.), *Handbook of clinical research* (pp. 31–60). Thousand Oaks, CA: Sage.

Watson, J. (1979). *Nursing: The philosophy and science of caring*. Boston, MA: Little, Brown.

Watson, J. (1999a). *Nursing: Human science and human care: A theory of nursing*. Sudbury, MA: Jones & Bartlett Learning.

Watson, J. (1999b). *Postmodern nursing and beyond.* London, UK: Churchill Livingstone.

Watson, J. (2008). *Nursing: The philosophy and science of caring* (rev. ed.). Boulder, CO: University Press of Colorado.

Zander, P. E. (2007). Ways of knowing in nursing: The historical evolution of a concept. *Journal of Theory Construction & Testing, 11*(1), 7–11.

CARITAS EDUCATION IN ACADEMIC SETTINGS

My Quest for Caritas Literacy

–Mark D. Beck, DNP, MSN, BS, RN-BC, CENP, certified HeartMath trainer, Watson Caring Science Institute postdoctoral fellow, Caritas Coach

M ark describes his caritas journey as moving from *doing* to *being*–first to embody Caring Science in himself, and then as a way to creatively prepare nurses for the 21st century. The caritas literacies of acceptance, belonging, connection, and empowerment shift the educational paradigm toward respect, honor, and co-creation of a caring curriculum that fosters the growth of caritas nurses.

MARK'S CARITAS JOURNEY

My journey to becoming a Caritas Coach was a watershed moment in my life and career. My then-employer had recently adopted Watson's Caring Science framework as its foundational theory for the delivery of inpatient nursing care. As director of the clinical education, practice, and informatics team for two hospitals, it was incumbent upon me to use Watson's framework in the orientation and nurturing of the nursing staff. I applied and was accepted into the Caritas Coach Education Program (CCEP)—thus began my quest for caritas literacy.

For me, caritas literacy has been an ontological process of becoming more of who I really am—experiencing an *embodied metanoia* and manifesting my authentic self (Watson, 2017). I say embodied metanoia because for as long as I can remember, I have lived in my head. I saw my body as merely a vehicle for my head. As for my heart, it rode shotgun to my head and body. What I have learned from the Caritas Coach program is to stop and really *feel* where in my body my emotions and responses reside. Caritas was not only a mental exercise. This transformation occurred in mind, body, and spirit.

According to Merriam-Webster (n.d.), *metanoia* comes from the Greek *meta noein*, meaning change in mindset. In classical Greek, the word's meaning was expanded to also suggest a change of heart. Today, the most common use of the word comes from the Biblical Greek meaning to transform through a turning back or repentance.

This process of learning to feel my emotions in my body was gradual and subtle. As I learned to become present—both with myself and others—I began to feel inklings of emotions in various places in my body. Like many working professionals, I typically carry my stress in my neck, shoulders, and lower back. I have even ruptured my lower lumbar area by carrying so much stress. But because I lived in my head and not in my body, I never felt my body talking to me about my stress level.

I think of it like a person riding an elephant. The rider has the illusion that he or she is in charge of the elephant. But the *real* power lies in the motivation and momentum of the elephant. To successfully ride the elephant, the rider must be one with the elephant, sensing its mood, fear, and motivation. In the same way I must be one with my body. To extend the metaphor, most change initiatives fail because they address only the cognitive structure of the rider, not the emotional state of the elephant (Heath & Heath, 2010).

Although the foundation of my transformation began in the Caritas Coach program, it did not fully blossom until after I suffered a heart attack. Only then did I actually begin to listen to my body for its messages. I now have begun to live in my body—not just my head. This transformation is most profound for me as I now see and feel the world and those in it differently. I listen with my eyes and see with my ears. I become an observant listener to find the heart of the matter. It has taken me some 55 years, but I can now be myself.

About 3 months after I completed the Caritas Coach program, I attended the annual holiday work party. My staff and I were performing an exercise in which we said what we appreciated about each other. The woman facilitating the exercise shared how grateful staff members were for my improved ability to listen to and appreciate them. Members of the staff then asked me to explain what had happened to me—they wanted to know what had changed. "I'm just more comfortable in my own skin," I explained. They asked for clarification. "It's like the story about how the rhinoceros got his skin in the *Just So Stories* by Rudyard Kipling," I said (Kipling, 1902). "I was able to take off my skin and shake out the cake crumbs in it that had been causing me to be irritable, short, mean, and dreadful."

At last, I was able to be in my skin, and it felt wonderful. Moreover, being more myself, I was able to listen with my heart and head, and to feel my responses in my body. This enabled me to be in right relation with my head, my heart, and the source, or universal love (Watson, 2008). I was able to breathe, center, and be mindful of the ethic of belonging (Levinas, 1969). And because I belonged, I was able to invite the other to belong, too. I could make myself available in the moment by being present, and in doing so, I could connect with the other and allow the other to be herself or himself. It was as simple as that.

Seeing and Engaging Differently

Caring Science has transformed my whole view of the world. I now see and theorize very differently and engage the world in a new way. For example, since my Caritas Coach training, I do not view the creation of curriculum from the same viewpoint of knowledge (cognitive), skills (psychomotor), and attitudes (values and beliefs)—or KSA—in the same way. I've learned that attitudes are the entryway to engaging the scholar in the adoption of the knowledge and skills.

My purpose is to engage others in a manner that allows them to be heard, to have a sense of connection (belonging), and to be valued for their contribution. I do this very consciously in my role as curriculum designer for an RN-to-BSN program. In this role, I help the faculty infuse the Caring Science framework into the curriculum. We spread the 10 Caritas Processes across five semesters, creating assignments that align with course objectives and processes. As I set the objectives for each course, I make explicit the intentions of the lesson, starting with the why (Sinek, 2011). The design faculty can then visualize the outcomes that have been established and use them as a guide for their lesson assignments.

The program teaches students the foundations of the Caring Science framework. To create the workforce of the future, the desired program outcomes for each student are as follows:

- Create a vision of themselves in the future of nursing.
- Find their voice so they can tell their stories (their own as well as their patients').
- Having completed the first two objectives, nurses will be able to own their practice.

These outcomes facilitate the journey of self-discovery with:

- Authentic presence
- Authentic listening
- Holding space for another
- Understanding and practicing caritas literacy

Being in right relation—in other words, aligning head, heart, and source (Watson, 2008)—is a never-ending journey. It requires constant work. Students explore how to use skills intrinsic to each human—self-reflection, developing empathy and compassion, and unique expressions of their caring behaviors—to become embodied metanoia in their own right. My purpose is to help them continue this journey so their resilience and skills grow to a sustainable level by the time of graduation. An environment in which students can flourish (through creativity, connection, and belonging) (Seligman, 2012) allows for the innate expression (*epigenetics*) of what it means to be a full human being (Wheatley, 2017).

CO-CREATING THE LEARNING ENVIRONMENT

I use the core concepts of the *unitary-transformative caring model* (Cowling, Smith, & Watson, 2008; Watson, 2010) in my work designing the RN-to-BSN curriculum. My purpose is to co-create, along with the students, an environment for working nurses by which they discover that they already practice some of these core concepts (specifically wholeness, consciousness, and caring) (Cowling et al., 2008). I introduce to them the language of the unitary-transformative model to describe the phenomenon of nursing. The fundamental change in my being enables me to use all ways of knowing (Dwyer & Revell, 2015) in my work. This allows me to create curriculum and co-create the learning environment to encourage further exploration of experiential learning and the core concepts of the theory.

Even though most of my students come from a health system that has Caring Science as its foundation, they have only an inkling of the true value and meaning of that framework. It is satisfying to watch them find their own voice and story, and begin to sense what it means to own their practice. Just 6 weeks into the curriculum, many students say they view their interactions with the patients in their care—and the patients' families—differently. They also enjoy better relationships with their peers.

Some of the hardest work these students do is the internal work of becoming a reflective practitioner (Johns, 2013). This work mirrors the work in mindfulness-based stress reduction (MBSR) (Kabit-Zin, 1991), which is part of the curriculum. All classes begin with a centering moment. Centering allows the faculty and students to create an internal and external environment that enables them to be authentically present in the class. Engagement and the degree to which students are willing to reveal their vulnerabilities have increased in all cohorts. As Brown puts it, vulnerability is the heart of joy, love, connection with self and other, and true belonging as well as pain, fear, and disconnection (2010, 2012, 2015, 2017). The depth of learning and transformation is made manifest in their evaluations and anecdotal encounters.

One student in the RN-to-BSN program provided evidence of such a transformation:

> During this semester, I learned to be open and vulnerable in all situations I encounter. This experience made me realize that throughout my career and my personal life I had an enormous amount of fear. [Caring Science] has opened my eyes to awareness of myself. Therefore, I could open myself up to others. This course has given me the tools to widen the lens that I view the world around me. Being exposed to Jean Watson's Caritas Processes during this program has changed my practice as a clinician. The Caritas Processes have also influenced my personal life...

One of the most impactful significant lessons in [Caring Science] was the unitary-transformative model. Being able to care for self and others' entire being. Allowing myself to be vulnerable in each moment and interaction with others. Before this program, my thought process was very one-directional. Looking back at my career and personal life I was narrow-minded. However, I did not realize it at the time. The tools given to me through the [Caring Science] course will stay with me my entire life. This course gave me the confidence to face my fears. I have shared the information I have learned with my coworkers, management, and family. The transformation within myself has changed the environment around me. The new ways of learning—for example, the mind map analysis—allowed me to learn important clinical information—that my practice was lacking—in a creative way. Once I faced my fears of learning in a new fashion and embraced the process, I really enjoyed the process. (Kolb, 2017)

HELPING NURSES FIND THEIR VOICE AND OWN THEIR PRACTICE

One strategy used to promote self-awareness and self-care, and to help students find their voice, is the use of vision boards. Vision boards help the student illustrate in picture form how they envision the future of nursing and how they fit in this vision. These student-created vision boards reveal a remarkable transformation in self-awareness and self-care and an expansion of the possibilities they envision for their career. Each student's vision board becomes part of his or her e-portfolio, which students create as part of their final project for the program.

Learning the language of Caring Science and exploring the unitary-transformative model (wholeness, consciousness, and caring) enable students to name their nursing phenomena—in particular, the art of nursing—and thus begin to own their practice. This is why we must be clear about the language we use in the discipline of nursing. The power of language comes from the act of naming and gives the speaker power over the concepts and phenomena (Graham, 2013). It enables the speaker of the name to own the concept. This is the secret to students learning to own their practice. With ownership comes empowerment. This quest of naming is how I have used the transformation in my own embodied metanoia to change the way I show up in my work and world, and how I've improved my own caritas literacy.

CONNECTING WITH SOURCE AND READING THE FIELD

My own reflective practice enables me to connect with source and envision new ways to engage. (By source, I mean how a person imagines he or she is connected to God, the universe, or a higher purpose. This is key to the sense-making function of the affective domain.) This activity is enhanced when I am in class and I read the room or the energy patterns that emerge from students. My self-awareness and my understanding of the intention of the lesson enable me to alter the direction and support of the lesson in the moment. I use film clips and music videos to illustrate concepts. These more effectively enable students to delve into their feelings around a topic than my words do. These strategies are caritas literacy in action—a way to tie caritas literacy to teaching strategies and ways of being and becoming.

Being in right relation (Watson, 2005) enables me to access a much deeper well of creativity than I could with just my own consciousness. Setting my intention for the work and bringing my head and heart into alignment using HeartMath techniques have exponentially increased my creativity. I have made it a practice to enter coherence—that is, to foster heart rhythm synchronicity between the heart and brain, known as *heart-rate variability* (HRV), which is an indicator of health and well-being (Childre & Cryer, 2000; Childre, Martin, Rozman, &

McCraty, 2016)—when I enter and leave a creative space. This practice enables me to access my previous creative endeavors and to shorten the time until the next one.

Educators are familiar with the use of Bloom's taxonomies in the preparation of their curricula. Nursing educators are especially gifted in the cognitive and psychomotor domains of learning—the domains stressed by most curricula. The *affective domain* is where values, attitudes, and beliefs engage with and motivate behaviors (Valiga, 2014). Much of curriculum development mirrors that of the basic sciences in medicine, pathophysiology, and pharmacology. These models are predicated upon the mechanistic view of the body, where the body has been deconstructed as a machine (Sheldrake, 2013). Possessing a growth mind set (Dweck, 2006) is key to success, and engaging the affective domain is essential to establishing a growth mindset.

HeartMath techniques include heart-focused breathing–that is, bringing the communication of the heart-brain into rhythmic communication that leads to coherence.

In creating the curriculum, I have developed what I call the *affective domain arc*. The affective domain enables sense-making or meaning-making for these values, beliefs, and attitudes. The arc refers to how the affective domain connects all aspects of learning—cognitive, psychomotor, and so on—in its function of sense-making (Madsbjerg, 2017). It enables me to create hooks on which cognitive and psychomotor information can hang. This arc decreases each student's cognitive load by enabling them to place the information on the hook that is most appropriate (Valiga, 2014). I have found that this technique helps students increase their retention of information, as the information now has a "home." Students tell me they "get it" (Taylor, 2014). Their evaluations and anecdotal encounters demonstrate the value of this approach.

As educators, we are familiar with knowledge, skills, and attitudes (KSAs) from the Quality and Safety Education for Nurses (QSEN) competencies (Sherwood & Barnsteiner, 2012). I have reframed this as KSA 2.0, or ASK (attitudes, skills, and knowledge). The values, beliefs, and attitudes—the realm of the affective domain—we all hold are the entryway to creating a hunger for the cognitive and psychomotor domains. They give context, which is why we should always start with *why* (Sinek, 2011).

FINAL REFLECTIONS

My quest for caritas literacy has led me to embodied metanoia, which has revolutionized my way of being and showing up in the world. It has allowed me to access a way of seeing and embody feeling in my own practice. My purpose is now to co-create environments for nurses to learn the language of the discipline of Caring Science in nursing, to find their voices so they can tell their story, and to then own their practice. By grounding themselves in their practice with resilience and emancipatory knowing (Chinn & Kramer, 2011; Watson & Smith, 2002), nurses ensure that in the future, nursing will be a vibrant cornerstone of the healthcare system—not only in their institutions but in their communities and globally as they serve humanity.

REFERENCES

Brown, B. (2010). *The gifts of imperfection.* Center City, MN: Hazelton.

Brown, B. (2012). *Daring greatly: How the courage to be vulnerable transforms the way we live, love, parent and lead.* New York, NY: Penguin Random House.

Brown, B. (2015). *Rising strong: How the ability to reset transforms the way we live, love, parent and lead.* New York, NY: Penguin Random House.

Brown, B. (2017). *Braving the wilderness: The quest for true belonging and the courage to stand alone.* New York, NY: Penguin Random House.

Childre, D., & Cryer, B. (2000). *From chaos to coherence: The power to change performance.* Boulder Creek, CA: HeartMath Inc.

Childre, D., Martin, H., Rozman, D., & McCraty, R. (2016). *Heart intelligence: Connecting with the intuitive guidance of the heart.* Cardiff, CA: Waterfront Digital Press.

Chinn, P., & Kramer, M. (2011). *Integrated theory and knowledge development in nursing* (8th ed.). London, UK: Elsevier.

Cowling, W. R. III, Smith, M. C., & Watson, J. (2008). The power of wholeness, consciousness, and caring: A dialogue on nursing science, art, and healing. *Advances in Nursing Science, 31*(1), E41–51. doi:10.1097/01. ANS.0000311535.11683.d1

Dweck, C. (2006). *Mindset: The new psychology of success.* New York, NY: Random House.

Dwyer, P. A., & Revell, S. M. H. (2015). Preparing students for the emotional challenges of nursing: An integrative review. *Journal of Nursing Education, 54*(1), 7–12. doi:10.3928/01484834-20141224-06

Graham, L. (2013). The power of names: In culture and in mathematics. *Proceedings of the American Philosophical Society, 157*(2), 229–234.

Heath, C., & Heath, D. (2010). *Switch: How to change things when change is hard.* New York, NY: Crown Business.

Johns, C. (2013). *Becoming a reflective practitioner* (4th ed.). Hoboken, NJ: Wiley-Blackwell.

Kabit-Zin, J. (1991). *Full catastrophe living.* New York, NY: Delta.

Kipling, R. (1902). How the rhinoceros got his skin. *Just So Stories.* London, UK: Macmillan.

Kolb, S. (2017). Personal communication.

Levinas, E. (1969). *Totality and infinity: An essay on exteriority.* Pittsburgh, PA: Duquesne University Press.

Madsbjerg, C. (2017). *Sensemaking: The power of the humanities in the age of the algorithm.* New York, NY: Little Brown.

Metanoia. (n.d.). *Merriam-Webster Online.* Retrieved from https://www.merriam-webster.com/dictionary/metanoia

Seligman, M. E. P. (2012). *Flourish: A visionary new understanding of happiness and well-being.* New York, NY: Free Press.

Sheldrake, R. (2013). *Set science free: 10 paths to new discovery.* New York, NY: Random House.

Sherwood, G., & Barnsteiner, J. (2012). *Quality and safety in nursing: A competency approach to improving outcomes.* Hoboken, NJ: John Wiley & Sons.

Sinek, S. (2011). *Start with why: How great leaders inspire everyone to take action.* New York, NY: Portfolio.

Taylor, L. D. (2014). *The affective domain in nursing education: Educators' perspectives.* University of Wisconsin Milwaukee. Retrieved from https://samuelmerritt. idm.oclc.org/login?url=http://search.ebscohost.com/login.aspx?direct=true&db=r zh&AN=109774671&site=ehost-live

Valiga, T. M. (2014). Attending to affective domain learning: Essential to prepare the kind of graduates the public needs. *Journal of Nursing Education, 53*(5), 247. doi:10.3928/01484834-20140422-10

Watson, J. (2005). Caring before belonging. *Nursing Science Quarterly, 18*(4), 302–303.

Watson, J. (2008). *Nursing: The philosophy and science of caring* (rev. ed.). Boulder, CO: University Press of Colorado.

Watson, J. (2010). Caring science and the next decade of holistic healing: Transforming self and system from the inside out. *Beginnings, 30*(2), 14–16.

Watson, J. (2017). *Global advances in human caring literacy*. New York, NY: Springer Publishing Co.

Watson, J., & Smith, M. C. (2002). Caring science and the science of unitary human beings: A trans-theoretical discourse for nursing knowledge development. *Journal of Advanced Nursing, 37*(5), 452–461.

Wheatley, M. J. (2017). *Who do we choose to be? Facing reality, claiming leadership, restoring sanity*. Oakland, CA: Berret-Koehler Publishers.

Living a Caritas Consciousness: A Philosophy for Our Everyday Practices as Nurse Educators

-Lisa Goldberg, PhD, RN, Caritas Coach

Lisa shares her caritas journey, and how she reclaimed the joy of teaching by learning and reimagining new possibilities in nursing education. In the Caritas Coach Education Program (CCEP), Lisa discovered that her intentional and conscious relationship with herself, and her transpersonal relationships with others, revitalized her vision as a compassionate, loving, accepting, and collaborative educator.

LISA'S CARITAS JOURNEY

"The transpersonal caring model incorporates soul care—fostering ongoing self-growth, spiritual growth and healing for the wounded healer." (Watson, 1999, p. 180)

In 2004, I graduated from the University of Alberta, Canada, with my PhD in nursing. Excited and determined to carve out my career as a new nurse educator and researcher, I returned home to Nova Scotia to take up an academic position at Dalhousie University School of Nursing. With a passionate commitment to the cultivation of scholarship that equally valued research, teaching, and clinical practice, I embodied my academic trajectory with purpose and enthusiasm for all that was possible in my new role.

As the years went on and institutional constraints—including the academy's emphasis of research over teaching and of grant capture and publication over education—became burdensome, I found myself disillusioned. I questioned my decision to continue as a nurse academic. This disillusionment soon became obvious due to my changing disposition toward those around me—including, regrettably, the students. Negative teaching evaluations soon reflected this change in me.

Despite the pain and self-doubt I experienced while reading these evaluations, they became a transformative tool for change. I realized I had to either leave my academic life and find an alternative profession or reclaim joy and reimagine possibilities beyond my current situation. After much self-reflection and inner dialogue, I chose joy, I chose love, and I chose forgiveness (Watson, 2008)—forgiveness of self, of others, and of a system that was often relentless and unforgiving.

Perhaps I was already channeling a caritas consciousness—one embodied in the philosophy of Caring Science developed by world-renowned nurse theorist Dr. Jean Watson (2008). As Watson (2005) reminds us:

> When we are so oriented toward control, domina-
> tion, with a sense of rational knowing that we are
> responsible for making things happen; the concept of
> surrendering is foreign to us and our ego world of op-
> eration. Nevertheless, it often is only through surren-
> dering, in letting go of ego—sense of control and our
> efforts to make something happen, that we witness
> new possibilities unfolding in front of us. (p. 118)

While the language of love, joy, and forgiveness is easily dismissed in academic settings, this was the very language that inspired
me on my new and transformative journey toward being and becoming caritas (Watson, 2008).

Through the Caritas Coach program, I discovered how to cultivate caritas literacy by living the 10 Caritas Processes. Grounded in
the philosophy of Caring Science (Goldberg, 2015; Watson, 2008),
this experiential and scholarly
journey revitalized my academic
vision by locating me in a caritas
consciousness—one that embodies a reflexive, compassionate, and
politically dynamic pedagogy for
our scholarship as nurse educators
(Goldberg, Rosenburg, & Watson,
2017).

While there are numerous definitions for
pedagogy, common to most is the view
that it provides a theoretical framework and
pragmatic application to inform teaching
and learning practices–that is, interactions,
judgments, strategies, and interventions.

TOWARD BEING AND BECOMING CARITAS

As my journey toward being and becoming caritas began, I found
myself searching for ways to more deeply embody my role as an educator and mentor to engage collaboratively with students. Reflecting on that time, I realize I was attempting to reclaim my heart as a

teacher—not only for myself, but also for the students with whom I was privileged to collaborate (Palmer, 2007).

Recognizing that my negative student evaluations were an opportunity for change, my initial search took me to the university's Centre for Learning and Teaching (CLT). I was privileged to begin a collegial relationship with Dr. Suzanne Le-May Sheffield, the director of CLT. Through our many dynamic conversations across a continuum of learning and teaching, pedagogical philosophies, and diversity, I soon came to understand the central role compassion plays in pedagogy where politicization is an overarching goal. In other words, as a teacher committed to an ontological approach to nursing as a politicized practice, compassion and love are necessary if the political is to be embraced by students as an everyday act (Goldberg, 2015; Watson, 2008). Perhaps hooks (2000) captures this best:

> …we accept that true love is rooted in recognition and acceptance, that love combines acknowledgment, care, responsibility, commitment, and knowledge, we understand there can be no love without justice. (p. 104)

Upon my recognition that compassion and love were necessary for students to understand how to cultivate a more politicized practice including, but not limited to, the relevance of social justice, health equity, and the advancement of underrepresented and underserved communities, I continued my journey toward caritas—one in which I more deeply committed to understanding the embodiment of the 10 Caritas Processes and how they could be lived on a daily basis as a Caritas Coach.

THE CARITAS COACH PROGRAM

In the spring of 2014, I began the CCEP, a transformative journey over a 6-month period through the Watson Caring Science Institute

(WCSI) in Boulder, Colorado. Surrounded by the majestic beauty of Boulder, which sits at the foothills of the Rocky Mountains, I embarked on a quest through on-site retreats, distance learning, scholarly reading and writing, and one-on-one mentorship with an exceptional WCSI faculty member, Dr. Lynne Wagner. This fostered an understanding of Caring Science through a form of caritas literacy grounded in the 10 Caritas Processes. This experiential and philosophical understanding illuminated how to inhabit the role of a Caritas Coach as a living, breathing extension of the self (Goldberg, 2015).

THE 10 CARITAS PROCESSES

Being and becoming a Caritas Coach is grounded in the 10 Caritas Processes. Collectively, these processes provide a framework that engages the practitioner in caritas literacy that can be applied in professional and personal practices.

Beginning with the reflexive self, the 10 Caritas Processes invite the practitioner to engage in a deep understanding of the self, before cultivating trusting and authentic relationships with others. Through the application of these processes—rooted in loving kindness, transparency, the development of a genuine commitment to teaching and learning, and the ability to cultivate a spiritual practice (including a belief in magic and miracles)—the practitioner cultivates caritas literacy (Watson, 2008). Thus, the 10 Caritas Processes collectively provide an action-oriented approach to guide practitioners (educator, clinician, administrator, and researcher) while cultivating an authentic, loving, spiritual, and transpersonal relationship with self, other, and the broader community (Goldberg, 2015; Watson, 2008).

Embodying one's role as a Caritas Coach can begin only when one moves beyond the ego-self (Goldberg, 2015; Watson, 2008). Thus it is only in the abandonment of ego that transpersonal caring can begin—that the practitioner (educator) in that moment can authentically begin to understand the inner world and storied life of the other (student). Watson (2010) eloquently characterizes transpersonal caring as an

> ...intersubjective, human-to-human relationship, which encompasses two individuals in a given moment, but simultaneously transcends the two, connecting to other dimensions of being and a deeper/higher consciousness that accesses the universal field and planes of inner wisdom: the human spirit. (p. 115)

Thus, transpersonal caring in the context of education suggests an opportunity on the part of the educator to be fully present with the student, providing the educator an authentic and rare opportunity to stay with the other's point of reference (Watson, 2010). In so doing, a new moment in time and space is co-created, transcending the experience of the one to the experience of the two together—educator and learner, teacher and student (Sitzman & Watson, 2013; Watson, 2010).

CARITAS LITERACY

As one learns to embody a caritas consciousness through the application of the 10 Caritas Processes—including an understanding of transpersonal caring (in which the educator authentically focuses on the student with a fullness of attention through concern, meaning, and love [Sitzman & Watson, 2013])—the ongoing cultivation of a unique way of being in the world is required. This results in caring literacy (Watson, 2008). As beautifully articulated by Watson (2008), this literacy includes

> ...an evolved and continually evolving emotional heart intelligence, consciousness and intentionality and level of sensitivity and efficacy, followed by a continuing lifelong process and journey of self-growth and self-awareness. Such an

awakening of one's being and abilities cultivates
skills and awareness of holding, conveying, and
practicing communicating thoughts of caring,
loving-kindness, equanimity, and so on as part of
one's professional Being. (p. 23)

This description suggests the nature of this work is ongoing and
forever in process. As a Caritas Coach, understanding how these
practices are cultivated professionally can assist practitioners in
recognizing the lived and action-oriented nature of this work. For
example, the practitioner does not simply engage with the environment "to make significant changes in ways of Being/doing/knowing"
(Watson, 2008, p. 26). Rather, the practitioner is considered to *be*
the environment in which the change is taking place. This becomes
an essential ingredient for the Caritas Coach who becomes a caritas
educator.

In becoming the environment that heals, caritas educators are
invited to share in the profound influences they have on the spaces
and places they inhabit (Watson, 2008). This results from their self-
reflexive and highly cultivated awareness regarding their own energy
field(s) and the ways in which this can radiate intentionality and
consciousness (Watson, 2005; Watson, 2008). This may positively or
negatively influence educational spaces, including those with students and faculty.

TEACHING AND LEARNING

The integration of caring literacy into my own teaching and learning practices while promoting an embodied commitment to dwell
with the experiences of others (Watson, 2008) is foundational to
my transformative success in my teaching-learning relationships
with students as a Caritas Coach. In what follows, I provide specific
examples of how this is lived in my everyday practices in the context
of my teaching.

CARING SCIENCE PEDAGOGY

Promoting a scholarly and critically stimulating environment for student engagement is essential to advancing excellence in future students at both the undergraduate and graduate level. I thus work to co-create a reflexive, compassionate, and politicized approach to my teaching and learning by using a pedagogical framework grounded in Caring Science. This organically aligns with feminist, queer, and phenomenological theories (Ahmed, 2006; Goldberg et al., 2017; Goldberg, 2015; Goldberg, Harbin, & Campbell, 2011; Goldberg, Ryan, & Sawchyn, 2009; Merleau-Ponty, 1965; Watson, 2008; Young, 2005). In other words, because Caring Science is epistemologically pluralistic, ontologically holistic, and ethically inclusive, it has the capacity to align with a diverse set of philosophical frameworks (Hills & Watson, 2011; Watson, 2008).

Collectively, these philosophies guide my educational pedagogy and reflect the following:

- Students are expert in their own storied experiences and provide legitimate forms of knowledge.

- Students and educators alike are positioned, albeit often unknowingly, in unforgiving systems plagued by a historical legacy of institutional discrimination (racism, sexism, homophobia, etc.). This reflects the starting point for the stories they tell and the experiences they live.

- As a self-reflexive educator (Goldberg, 2015), I aim to cultivate authentic, reciprocal, trusting, and compassionate relationships with students, faculty, and others within my academic community (Hills & Watson, 2011; Watson, 2008).

- By integrating the aforementioned within a Caring Science pedagogy, I invite self-reflexivity with students, thus potentiating understanding in what it means to be a compassionate, politically astute, and ethically sensitive clinician in the broadest sense in today's healthcare system (Goldberg, 2015).

CREATING A SPACE

Creating a space that is open, safe, relational, and respectful for all students is vital to optimizing learning (Hills & Watson, 2011). Few can blossom in educational environments that are unsupportive. Recently, I have engaged in new approaches that are positioned within the "dimensions of caring literacy" (Watson, 2008, p. 25) when collaborating with students. For example, at the onset of a clinical practicum, I now invite students to engage in a discussion of learning and teaching styles, including my own. This has enabled students to reflect more deeply on how they learn best and in turn how I can best support them in their clinical learning. This has allowed me to cultivate a more mindful caring consciousness (Watson, 2008) in my teaching and learning practices, in addition to understanding the diverse challenges many students face in the context of their learning.

A learning space that connotes healing, trust, and authenticity with and for students can be created through a variety of methods and can be consistently aligned within a pedagogy grounded in Caring Science (Hills & Watson, 2011; Watson, 2008). Drawing on my daily practices as a Caritas Coach, I have been inspired to integrate my personal and professional practices into the graduate nursing philosophy course I redesigned and currently teach. The 3-hour seminar, which is grounded in Caring Science, introduces students to diverse theories in nursing and philosophy. Currently it commences with a meditation, a circle formation, and a weekly ritual of tea. As Okakura (1919) so poetically reminds us:

> Teaism is a cult founded on the adoration of the beautiful among the sordid facts of everyday existence. It inculcates purity and harmony, the mystery of mutual charity, the romanticism of the social order. It is essentially a worship of the imperfect, as it is a tender attempt to accomplish something possible in this impossible thing we know as life. (pp. 3–4)

The ritual of tea sharing is new to students. After all, the standard graduate class does not traditionally involve the professor arriving with a tea trolley and numerous pots of flavored teas. Although the teas may vary from week to week, the outcome is always the same: robust, inspirational, and lively discussion. The simple gesture of introducing tea to the classroom space as a weekly experience unites the class and creates a relaxed and trusting environment for philosophical and experiential conversation. As one student wrote in the signed evaluative comments from the student ratings of instruction carried out by the University Centre for Learning and Teaching:

> Lisa...has a very calming presence and began each class with not only pots of tea but also an allotted amount of time for us all to go around and share our thoughts based on the week's readings/theme and how they related to our practice areas...She was available outside of class and very prompt in returning course communication...It was great to learn from her recent journey in Caring Science as well and learn from the guest speakers she invited to class—all of whom were wonderful. (n. p.)

These comments were reflective of the class evaluations. The tea ritual assisted in creating a learning environment in which trust, safety, and relationships flourished. As such, it has become a standard feature of the course.

THE ACT OF LISTENING

Active listening that has been collaboratively informed by constructive feedback from students is essential to understanding their experiential frame of reference (Watson, 2008). Hills and Watson (2011) suggest

> ...listening is the most important process in
> critical caring dialogue, and it is at the heart of an

emancipatory relational curriculum. Without effective listening, dialogue is reduced to mere words. We
can begin to engage in the crucial caring dialogue
only through understanding another's meaning.
(p. 88)

The act of listening provides another example of how to cultivate
Caring Science pedagogy by living one's caritas literacy through the
application of the 10 Caritas Processes. Further, "empathic listening requires not only that we hear what is being said but also that
we respond in ways that demonstrate that we understood another's
meaning" (Hills & Watson, 2011, p. 89). In addition to active and
empathic listening, I make myself readily available to students via
email, and mindfully respond to correspondence within 24 hours. I
have an open door policy for office hours and am always delighted
to see students in person, via appointment or by chance. Engaging with students in this way promotes their confidence and trust
in my communication abilities as an educator. Finally, I am quick
to learn names, and I work diligently to commit them to memory. I
also consider eye contact as appropriate to culture and circumstance
(Watson, 2008). To know the name of the other connotes familiarity,
creates trust, and fosters engagement.

FINAL REFLECTIONS

My caritas journey has profoundly evolved since my initial visit to
CLT. Through my Caritas Coach training, my approach as an educator, researcher, and scholar has evolved in ways I never imagined
possible. Understanding the necessary connection between compassion and politics through self-reflexivity within a Caring Science pedagogy for nursing is perhaps one of my greatest discoveries. It feeds
my soul and fosters a reclaimed generosity in my everyday practices.
Perhaps most importantly, I have returned to the heart of my teaching (Palmer, 2007) with renewed joy for all that is possible, much as
I did upon arriving at the university in 2004.

I have imperfect days when my caritas consciousness doesn't rise to the level of generosity, compassion, or forgiveness I expect—not only for students but also for myself. Still, I have a renewed ability to approach the classroom with politics and compassion for all that is possible in the nurses of tomorrow. For as hooks (1994) so powerfully writes:

> The academy is not a paradise. But learning is a place where paradise can be created. The classroom, with all its limitations, remains a location of possibility. In that field of possibility, we have the opportunity to labor for freedom, to demand of ourselves and our comrades an openness of mind and heart that allows us to face reality even as we begin to move beyond the boundaries, to transgress. (p. 2007)

REFERENCES

Ahmed, S. (2006). *Queer phenomenology: Orientations, objects, others.* Durham, NC: Duke University Press.

Goldberg, L. (2015). Cultivating inclusivity with caring science in the area of LGBTQ education: The self-reflexive educator. *Faculty Focus, 23*(3), 15–17.

Goldberg, L., Harbin, A., & Campbell, S. (2011). Queering the birthing space: Phenomenological interpretations of the relationships between lesbian couples and perinatal nurses in the context of birthing care. *Sexualities, 14,* 173–192.

Goldberg, L., Rosenburg, N., & Watson, J. (2017). Rendering LGBTQ+ visible in nursing: Embodying the philosophy of caring science. *Journal of Holistic Nursing,* June. doi:10.1177/0898010117715141

Goldberg, L., Ryan, A., & Sawchyn, J. (2009). Feminist and queer phenomenology: A framework for perinatal nursing practice, research, and education for advancing lesbian health. *Healthcare for Women International, 30*(6), 536–549.

Hills, M., & Watson, J. (2011). *Creating a caring science curriculum: An emancipatory pedagogy for nursing.* New York, NY: Springer Publishing Co.

hooks, b. (1994). *Teaching to transgress: Education as the practice of freedom.* Abington, UK: Routledge.

hooks, b. (2000). *Feminism is for everybody: Passionate politics.* London, UK: Pluto Press.

Merleau-Ponty, M. (1965). *The phenomenology of perception* (C. Smith, Trans.). Abington, UK: Routledge. (Original work published 1945).

Okakura, K. (1919). *The book of tea.* Carlisle, MA: Applewood Books. (Original work published 1906).

Palmer, P. J. (2007). *The courage to teach: Exploring the inner landscape of a teacher's life* (10th ed.). Hoboken, NJ: John Wiley & Sons.

Sitzman, K., & Watson, J. (2013). *Caring science, mindful practice: Implementing Watson's human caring theory.* New York, NY: Springer Publishing Co.

Watson, J. (1999). *Postmodern nursing and beyond.* London, UK: Churchill Livingstone.

Watson, J. (2005). *Caring science as sacred science.* Philadelphia, PA: F. A. Davis Co.

Watson, J. (2008). *Nursing: The philosophy and science of caring* (rev. ed.). Boulder, CO: University Press of Colorado.

Watson, J. (2010). Caring science and the next decade of holistic healing: Transforming self and system from the inside out. *Beginnings, 30*(2), 14–16.

Young, I. M. (2005). *On female body experience: "Throwing like a girl" and other essays.* Oxford, UK: Oxford University Press.

CREATING AN ESSENCE OF COMPASSION: A PERSONAL REFLECTION ON THE JOURNEY THROUGH CARING SCIENCE

–JILL GARABED-HRUSKA, BSCN, CAE, CARITAS COACH

A nurse educator, Jill shares her experience as she moved toward a more conscious life and practice through embodiment of the caritas literacies. The foundation of her journey includes the practice of compassion and vulnerability, breathing into emotion, learning from life lessons, and a commitment to self-care. She in turn has been able to coach students on the use of mindfulness, meditation, and self-care to instill Caring Science in their own nursing practices.

JILL'S CARITAS JOURNEY

Every journey begins somewhere. My journey to becoming a Caritas Coach began with feelings of frustration and helplessness in my profession.

As an instructor in a practical nursing program, I was deeply troubled as I witnessed the art of nursing becoming overshadowed by a primary biomedical model of nursing. When I began my nursing career, holistically and compassionately caring for each patient was deeply ingrained. But now it seemed practice areas were chaotic and short-staffed, with cultures largely set by individuals who were spread too thin, and were tired and burned out. This influenced how nursing students were treated—not only by other nurses but also by instructors. I knew the pendulum had to swing back to balance the science of nursing with the lost art of nursing, but the likelihood of that happening seemed slim.

In the summer of 2015, my colleagues and I attended a 2-day in-service staff retreat on Caring Science. After participating in the retreat, I knew I needed to learn more, so I enrolled in the Caritas Coach Education Program (CCEP) that fall. My life would never be the same! Caring Science provided a framework to integrate the art and science of nursing by bringing a compassionate practice philosophy to the classroom and the bedside. Caring Science echoed what I already knew—I had simply lacked the language to share these beliefs and values with others. This enabled me to refocus my teaching and learning philosophy so that it centered on compassion.

For me, one key takeaway was realizing that the people I think are making my life miserable are actually hurting on the inside. I do not need to take it personally because it is never about me. More importantly, these people offer me an opportunity to grow. According to Watson (2008), we learn from others how to be more human by identifying ourselves with others and finding their dilemmas in ourselves. This concept changed the way I perceived everything. It was instrumental in setting the direction of my life and my practice. I am no longer a helpless victim of circumstance, but rather a centered observer of the miracle of life.

A DEEP REFLECTIVE JOURNEY

For me, becoming a Caritas Coach has been a deeply reflective journey into the science of compassion and caring. The ontology of Caring Science provides a nonlinear pathway of uncovering and cultivating the true nature of who we are as humans. Becoming submersed in and practicing the human caring theory provides the Caritas Coach with a map, language, and tools to live life authentically. Personal and professional practices align, transforming the way of being, relating, and connecting. A humbleness and vulnerability emerges that lends itself to deeper connections with people, experiences, and nature. This minimizes barriers and results in relationships that are more meaningful and fulfilling.

As children, human beings are resilient and open, inclusive and loving. But after experiencing pain, shame, and hurt, we often build walls and wear masks. This seems to reduce our chances of being hurt, but in reality creates a barrier that disguises our beautiful humanity and leaves us feeling isolated and disconnected. We begin to believe that we are lonely and separate from others. Humans are social and tribal creatures. We are healthier and better balanced when we have multiple social contacts and loving relationships. To live holistically and to meet our own needs, we must be able to connect with and trust each other. Trusting means removing our masks and deconstructing the walls we have built to protect ourselves.

Learning to be vulnerable again was one of the most difficult teachings for me as a Caritas Coach. Part of becoming vulnerable means redefining personal boundaries. To truly know myself and to create a compassionate essence, I had to allow myself to become vulnerable and transparent. Being vulnerable may seem frightening at first but as we begin to peel back the layers, we provide a gift to ourselves and to those we encounter. It is through this shedding of layers that we begin to remove the barriers that cause perceived separation and impair us in our ability to connect with our own humanity. It was only after I accepted my own vulnerability as a coach that I was able to truly practice the 10 Caritas Processes.

LEARNING TO NURTURE OURSELVES

Because our workplaces (and the world) often feel hectic and unsafe, boundaries are essential for the Caritas Coach. Boundaries enhance self-awareness and act as a point of reference to ensure that self-care is sustained. Through boundaries, we reveal who we truly are while simultaneously creating a buffer between experiences, places, or people that drain us. It is imperative to identify and understand both the cause of this energy drain and what it feels like when energy resources require replenishing. The map of emotions—having self-awareness of your emotional patterns—may help guide the coach in developing a point of reference that indicates it is time to retreat, relax, reflect, and recharge.

The first Caritas Process (Caritas Process 1) supports the philosophy of loving-kindness, compassion, and equanimity for self and others—otherwise referred to as *self-care* (Watson, 2008). It's the primary lesson of the caritas journey. To be a Caritas Coach, alignment with Caritas Process 1 is nonnegotiable. We must regularly and consistently practice self-care.

Self-care is particularly critical to combating compassion fatigue, which often results when caregivers fail to acknowledge that they must also be cared for. As stated by Sorenson, Bolick, Wright, and Hamilton (2016), "self-care was reported to be the most significant preventative measure [healthcare providers] could take to protect themselves from developing [compassion fatigue]" (p. 462). To successfully combat compassion fatigue, Caritas Coaches must equip themselves with tools that allow for spiritual, physical, and emotional rejuvenation. This is achieved through self-care practices such as meditation, practicing gratitude, showing forgiveness, and demonstrating equanimity (Watson, 2008). The coaching and mentoring I received during the CCEP encouraged me to deeply reflect on which of my needs were or were not being met, and to learn the importance of mending wounds in myself before mending the wounds of others.

Often, nurses new to Caring Science quickly realize they are innately better at caring for others than caring for themselves. Not surprisingly, they also report feeling angry, powerless, burned out, and frazzled from carrying the burdens of others. This is often compounded for nurses who have experienced trauma in their own lives—common among members of helping professions like nursing (Conti-O'Hare, 2002). If, however, these nurses can transform from the "walking wounded" to become what many call "wounded healers," they can use their personal experience of suffering to help build therapeutic relationships with others (Christie & Jones, 2014).

Sometimes my mind is like a cage of screaming monkeys, with few fleeting breaks in thought. How can we silence our mind and stem the tide of false realities to create space for mindful thought and reflection? The answer lies in learning to identify triggers and to appreciate the best areas of healing and reflection.

UNDERSTANDING OUR EMOTIONS

Like the olfactory feelers on a butterfly's antennae, emotions enable humans to sense the space and environment around them. Feelings act as meteorological navigators of our current state of being. They provide tangible sensory feedback. This enables us to ask questions like the following:

- Am I safe?
- Am I being threatened?
- Am I uncomfortable?
- Is there something I need to learn from this situation?

Feelings act as the meter by which we gauge growth opportunities. By allowing these feelings to enter into our bellies, hearts, and minds, we expand our consciousness and are led toward a place of peace and happiness. Even experiences perceived as irritants or annoyances allow us to expand our consciousness because all emotions teach us a lesson. According to Buddhist practices, whatever you're feeling, if you can breathe it in deeply and acknowledge others who experience the same emotions, you can create compassion (Chödrön, 1994). If I can breathe in anger in its entirety, meditating on the emotion during my inhalation, I can exhale compassion for all who have ever felt anger and in doing so release my anger.

Although we must accept our emotions into our consciousness as opportunities for compassion, we must ensure that we do not judge them as "good" or "bad." Nor must we fixate on them. If we do, they will become concrete within our reality (Chödrön, 1994). Acknowledge the emotion but do not label it. Simply allow it to drift in and out of the consciousness as a cloud drifts in the sky. Being authentically present with emotions and feelings decreases our tendency to solidify judgment and expectations of ourselves and others. Emotions are subjective ways to read and perceive the energy field and need not be judged as positive or negative.

For me, discovering this new way of understanding emotions changed everything. Breathing became the alchemy to enter the space that is desirable in Caring Science. It is the space, identified in Caritas Process 10, where miracles can occur. Breathing consciously opens the space for hope, faith, and all possibilities. Discovering conscious breathing was pivotal in my personal growth in Caring Science. I went from being reactive to being receptive, from defensive to diplomatic, and developed a level of knowing that created sacredness and faith.

Having a responsive heart and diplomatic mind feels wiser and safer than having a reactive heart and a defensive mind. We must understand, accept, and embrace that people are on their own journeys. When we feel defensive, we must recognize that others are not deliberately vindictive toward us. Rather, we are responding to the heightened emotional state of others experiencing stress in our presence. When we recognize this, we can become energy that adds value to the space and lives of all we encounter, creating enlightenment and compassion within the shared environment rather than feeding into the wounding energy.

It was within the vulnerability that occurs with the removal of protective masks and barriers that I opened my heart and felt in my belly the gifts that were bestowed upon me through deep and meaningful reflective encounters and relationships. Recognizing the freedom that comes with detaching from emotions enabled me to enter into a new, calmer personal space and bestow a quieter, more peaceful essence upon those with whom I share my field. Each day when I wake, I practice gratitude and recommit to the caritas practice with this thought:

> Today I set my intention to project the essence of beauty and compassion to the spaces and lives around me.

BEING PATIENT WITH SELF AND OTHERS

Some people experience important landmarks in their personal journeys at different times and places. Other people feel tired, worn, afraid, or victimized by society, coworkers, or their families. Many people are unable to grasp that their environment is affected by what's going on inside each person within it.

We all have people in our lives that trigger us emotionally. We all can give personal testimony to those toxic people in our lives who cause us emotional turmoil. We become convinced that if they could just disappear, our lives would be magically transformed. Often, these are people we love. Maybe a loved one suffers from addiction or a mood disorder. Or maybe they're simply in the midst of a challenging stage of growth and development. In my own life, I have often felt frustrated or angered by the behaviors of others. I have often been indignant that an individual could be so unaware, so difficult, and so mean to those around them. In the past I also had a habit of telling myself stories based on what I had interpreted my surroundings to be. These stories often triggered unnecessary frustration and stress.

In difficult relationships and situations, I have learned to practice patience. In this way, I can create opportunities for self-growth. As with emotions, all relationships and situations offer self-growth opportunities. Often, when the lessons are learned and absorbed, we can transcend difficult situations and the people associated with them.

While reflecting on the virtues of being a Caritas Coach, I discovered that for me, the key to compassion was patience with self and others. During the CCEP, while exploring this theory, I focused on an individual in my workplace that caused me much anger and grief. My mentor suggested I identify and feel the emotion I was experiencing, breathe in that emotion, and then send the person that sparked the emotion thoughts of compassion. It was a powerful exercise in how conscious breathing combined with compassion could change my perception and open the space to other possibilities. That single experience changed my life. Emotions perceived as negative could be viewed as painful and uncomfortable. But when I was willing to breathe in the emotion with inspiration and exhale equanimity, my perceptions began to change. I was able to practice patience for who and what the person was. Through patience and compassion, I could release the negative emotions and remove them from my reality.

A TRANSFORMATIVE PROCESS

Becoming a Caritas Coach has transformed my reflective process. I now see difficult situations as opportunities for growth. I also see that when a difficult emotion does not resolve itself within 90 seconds, it is because a reactive story has attached itself to my conscious thoughts. It is through recognition that a period of compassion is necessary that the situation transforms into a lesson.

When faced with situations that might once have been devastating or caused me to feel derailed, I can now reorient myself into a place of peace by providing care and compassion for myself. Jean Watson calls this *repatterning* (Watson, 2007, p. 134). Every painful experience brings with it a little bit of grit that polishes my spiritual self. In this way, my inner essence takes on the characteristics of a pearl. As a Caritas Coach, it sometimes seems the journey is difficult and redundant. But this repatterning—like the process producing a pearl—is necessary. Suffering is part of the human condition. When we perceive suffering as a gift, it becomes a pathway to deeper meaning.

ONGOING REFLECTIVE PRACTICE

Even after becoming trained in caritas, I recognized that meditation alone was not enough. I needed some other way to shift my awareness and move my emotions. I decided to use prayer beads. Rather than using the beads for prayer, however, I decided to use them to practice slow methodical breathing. With each breath, I slowly advanced my thumb along the strand of beads, massaging each one. I found that whatever emotion I was experiencing at the time literally dissipated. After several months of this practice, I realized I could use strong and difficult emotions to expand my experience and humanity. By allowing the experience and feelings to happen while remaining free of judgment, I could develop a deeper and more compassionate presence with and around myself. According to Watson (2008), when we nurture compassion in ourselves, we give birth to our deepest humanity and can show compassion and love to those we care for personally and professionally.

After completing the Caritas Coaching program, I became aware that I am a highly empathic person. This realization was very significant. A number of nurses may possess this characteristic, yet are unaware of it. As a result, they unknowingly take on other people's emotions and issues, mistaking them for their own. I now understand how I am often affected by the emotions of others. When students I teach feel anxious, fearful, or stressed, those feelings can affect me physically if I am not aware of the need to center and perform self-care. According to Akerjordet and Severinsson (2008), learning to perceive, express, and manage both personal emotions and the emotions of others is central to the development of leadership competencies that promote emotional and intellectual growth. One way to defuse feelings of anxiety, fear, or irritability among nursing students in the classroom or clinical setting is to include the practice of play, laughter, and wonder in self-care. Playfulness provides the Caritas Coach with one more way to create ripples of joy into the field of consciousness. By inviting joy and laughter, we can move energy faster. Consider how you might use play, joy, and laughter while mentoring or coaching. One way is to show short videos of babies or animals. These tend to amuse all, regardless of age, culture, or language.

During my initial months of reflection, while immersed in the theory of Caring Science in CCEP, certain themes kept resurfacing. I would experience weeks of joy and bliss thanks to self-care and reflection exercises. But then some old issue would rear its ugly head and I would quickly revert to my old ways, becoming angry, defensive, fearful, and reactive. I would begin to shut down. This left me feeling discouraged and defeated. I had expected that once an issue had been dealt with, it would be laid to rest—not continue to resurface into my psyche at inconvenient times. Revisiting and re-experiencing the same conflicts and challenges seemed redundant and harmful.

I voiced my frustration about this to a close colleague and friend. "Why is this popping up again?" I cried. "I thought it was behind me!" Her response triggered a huge epiphany for me. She said our lives are like a labyrinth. The labyrinth is a metaphor for what is sacred in our lives. Through its twists and turns and expansive nature, we are given the space to explore life in a nonlinear manner. And although the experiences of sorrow, heartache, guilt, regret, and shame may reoccur, so too do the experiences of joy and bliss. This serves as a reminder of the sacred heartbeat of life. (Similarly, becoming a Caritas Coach is not a linear path. The issues we struggle with repeat. Still, with patience and faith, these struggles will begin to change.)

Each time we revisit and reflect on experiences, we have the op-portunity to practice Caritas Process 2: being authentically present with ourselves so we may then be authentically present with others. Time in the labyrinth calms our minds and enables us to cultivate our own spiritual practice. When we accept that experiences will re-surface and will overwhelm and discourage us, we have an opportu-nity to feel the emotions, breathe into them, write about them, look for metaphors, and meditate on them. We develop deeper meaning and understanding in our own experiences. We create space inside ourselves. Each time they resurface we recognize them as old friends providing us with an opportunity to truly understand our humanity. The best way to relax into this somewhat terrifying (and other times delicious) experience we call life is to breathe deeply and surrender. Surrender into the difficulties of life and allow your higher wisdom to chart and navigate the course of the outcome.

MODELING THE WAY

Life experiences can leave us feeling exposed, vulnerable, and disconnected. To be a successful Caritas Coach, one must immerse oneself in the theories of Caring Science and coach others to do the same.

Here's an example from my own personal experience. I have observed that nursing students often experience great stress and anxiety before skills testing, during exams, and in clinical situations. This leaves them in a fight-or-flight state. I wanted to help them deal with this primal stress reaction. A colleague and I decided to help students create their own beaded bracelets, similar to the prayer beads I had been using. We provided them with a variety of beads to choose from and showed them how to craft the bracelets. Then we showed them how to use the bracelets in the practice of conscious breathing when faced with anxiety or stress. The idea was to teach students to focus on the pace and depth of their breath to help them refocus their attention and calm down.

First, we taught them to identify when they felt anxious or stressed and to recognize the signs of the fight-or-flight response. Then we instructed them to stop the task they were performing and use a slow, deep mindful breathing technique called *bhramari pranayama* to elicit a parasympathetic response. This technique begins with a full exhalation through the mouth while making a *whoosh* sound. The next step is to close one's eyes and silently inhale through the nose for a count of four and hold the breath for a count of seven. Finally, exhale through the mouth with a *whoosh* sound for a count of eight. This breath cycle is repeated for a total of four breaths. This breathing technique decreases respiratory, heart, and blood-pressure rates (Pramanik et al., 2009).

Over the next several weeks, students kept journals to record their experiences before, during, and after practicing conscious breathing. The results were remarkable. They reported that the beads, used in combination with breathing, created feelings of calmness, peace, and relaxation. Test anxiety decreased. The sympathetic nervous system's fight-or-flight response was managed and controlled. As a result, students could practice the theory of Caring Science in their own frame of reference.

Final Reflections

The Caritas Coach must acknowledge and accept the fragilities in our existing systems and institutions (even as we work to change them). The mission of the Caritas Coach is to teach all students, including nursing students, how to manage stress and handle all types of emotions. We must empower others by providing safe environments, managing and refocusing fear and stress in ourselves, reigniting the light of possibilities, and searching for the beauty in health and healing. We must acknowledge and focus on our tribal nature and recognize that we do best when we share our power to recharge our spirits, hearts, and communities. When we are present, loving, and compassionate, we are more likely to work collaboratively and demonstrate consciousness. We understand that we are not separate, but rather a collective body. Everything we say and do matters not only to ourselves but to all others. This is the path to being a successful Caritas Coach and a leader in Caring Science.

REFERENCES

Akerjordet, K., & Severinsson, E. (2008). Emotionally intelligent nurse leadership: A literature review study. *Journal of Nursing Management, 16*(5), 565–577. doi: 10.1111/j.1365-2834.2008.00893.x

Chödrön, P. (1994). *Start where you are: A guide to compassionate living.* Boulder, CO: Shambhala Publications.

Christie, W., & Jones, S. J. (2014). Lateral violence in nursing and the theory of the nurse as wounded healer. *Online Journal of Issues in Nursing, 19*(1), 5.

Conti-O'Hare, M. (2002). *The nurse as wounded healer: From trauma to transcendence.* Sudbury, MA: Jones and Bartlett Publishers.

Pramanik, T., Sharma, H. O., Mishra, S., Mishra, A., Prajapati, R., & Singh, S. (2009). Immediate effect of slow pace bhastrika pranayama on blood pressure and heart rate. *Journal of Alternative and Complementary Medicine, 15*(3), 293–295. doi:10.1089/acm.2008.0440

Sorenson, C., Bolick, B., Wright, K., & Hamilton, R. (2016). Understanding compassion fatigue in healthcare providers: A review of current literature. *Journal of Nursing Scholarship, 48*(5), 456–465. doi:10.111/jnu.12229

Watson, J. (2007). Watson's theory of human caring and subjective living experiences: Carative factors/caritas processes as a disciplinary guide to the professional nursing practice. *Texto & Contexto—Enfermagem, 16*(1), 129–135.

Watson, J. (2008). *Nursing: The philosophy and science of caring* (rev. ed.). Boulder, CO: University Press of Colorado.

CARITAS COACH: A WORK IN PROGRESS

–KATHLEEN S. OMAN, PHD, RN, FAEN, FAAN, CARITAS COACH

Kathy's story emphasizes her evolutionary journey as a seasoned educator as she dedicated herself to integrating Caring Science into doctoral-level education. She shares her inner experience of seeking caritas literacy and explores how to best support the development of its mastery in students and colleagues alike. Through exercises and examples of learning activities, Kathy demonstrates how she engages others in critical reflection to deepen learning and living in a way that affirms and sustains humanity.

KATHY'S CARITAS JOURNEY

Although the Caritas Coach Education Program (CCEP) is an excellent deep dive into caritas literacy, it is the continual practice of the 10 Caritas Processes and my personal self-care activities that sustain and cultivate it. Even as I use the title of Caritas Coach, I feel like I am still becoming one. My knowledge and understanding of caritas is ever-expanding. New insights continually shift how I see myself and how I interact in the world. My personal growth and awareness have affirmed my worldview that we all share our space, we all are responsible for each other, and we all need love and compassion.

The first aspect of becoming a Caritas Coach is very personal. I am now much more at ease with myself and others. I practice loving-kindness, compassion, and equanimity with *me*. And because I start with me, I'm able to do the same with others. My sense of peace and gratitude has deepened and flourished. Even the language I use is changing, particularly in my writing. (It takes me longer to find the right caring language in my verbal interactions, perhaps because of the immediate nature of conversation.) I am now more at ease using the words *love, beauty, mystery,* and *faith*—words that vibrate at a higher level and convey my sense of belonging, being, and becoming (Watson, 2008).

At the International Caritas Consortium Conference in Boston in 2016, the keynote speaker was Andy Bradley, founder of Frameworks 4 Change. The mission of this organization is to create and sustain consistently compassionate caring environments. During his address, Bradley told the audience to "fall in love with this moment because it will never happen again" (Bradley, 2016). I hold this beautiful sentiment and reflect on it frequently. We are here on Earth for such a short time; we all need to learn to make the most of it. I am especially reminded of this now, having suffered significant personal losses over the past few months: an aunt, my mother-in-law (who died on my birthday), and two very special dogs. My love, memories, and the many wonderful images of them that flash across my computer screen are all that are left of them. I am so grateful for these reminders.

Modeling the Way

I see myself as a role model for caritas and others see me that way, too. Indeed, people in my work settings expect me to *be* caritas.

But this is not always easy.

I have a colleague with whom I don't communicate very well. In my old pattern of behavior, I would probably just chalk this up to being on separate pages and continue to have poor interactions. Obviously, this would not foster any movement in our relationship or improve our ability to work together. Now, with my caritas training, I realize that although I can't change the way she communicates, I can find a way to successfully interact with and respond to her. Using my Caritas Coach ways of being, doing, and knowing—practicing loving-kindness, compassion, and equanimity; being authentically present; and being sensitive to self and others—I grow in caritas literacy practices and I remain mindful that my communications must be authentic and honest. I try to see her as being "just like me," to find ideas or issues on which we agree, and build from there.

These caritas strategies were put to the test with this colleague when, while working on a project together, it became evident that we have different work styles—I like to have a plan; she takes a more last-minute approach. Although we both reach an acceptable endpoint, we get there very differently. But instead of dwelling in my dread, I reminded myself that she was "just like me." We both wanted to get the work done and produce a quality product. I kept an open mind and held space for different ways of being and doing. In the end, we worked well together and produced a good product. By framing my own thoughts and attitudes in the affirmative, I helped create a positive experience.

PRACTICING SELF-AWARENESS USING CARITAS PROCESSES

The 10 Caritas Processes have become central in my thinking and my practice. Using these processes, I have shifted from a place of reaction and self-doubt to one of mindfulness and authenticity, largely by becoming more self-aware. To quote Jean Watson, "Self-awareness or self-knowledge is recognizing us in others, finding their dilemma in ourselves; the self we learn about…is every self, the universal human self" (Watson, 1999, p. 117; Watson, 2008, p. 81). Once we recognize our interconnectedness, we avoid reducing another person to an object. The reflective practices in the CCEP were the main cause of this increased self-awareness—particularly the time I spent writing my online posts. I wrote two of these posts each week. One was part of a group discussion read by other Caritas Coach students. The other was ready only by my coach/facilitator. These posts required a significant level of self-reflection about personal and professional experiences.

Four Caritas Processes resonate most strongly with me in my professional role as an educator:

- **Having authentic presence:** This takes the form of listening with my heart and really hearing the other person.

- **Understanding and working from another's frame of reference:** This is a requirement in the Caritas Coach role. Individuals will generate solutions or ideas for themselves. The Caritas Coach is there simply to support and encourage.

- **Approaching teaching and learning from a relation stance:** This changes the dynamic from one in which the teacher wields authority and knowledge over the student to one in which the teacher and student share authority and knowledge with one another. In other words, the teacher and student learn together and from each other.

- **Allowing for multiple ways of knowing:** This means allowing students to tap into nontraditional ways of learning. Creativity is celebrated and encouraged, and each student's perspective is respected and valued.

Compassionate Affirmations

One nurse in my CCEP cohort introduced us to a website called the Avatar Compassion Project (https://theavatarcourse.com/the-compassion-project-eng.html). Its mission is to increase the amount of compassion in the world. As the site says, "The solution that we've been looking for is more alignment and cooperation, more attention on service to others. We need to become citizens for the planet" (Palmer, n.d.). In other words, to quote Andy Bradley of Frameworks 4 Change, we need to shift from "ego to eco" (Bradley, 2016).

One exercise in particular from the Avatar Compassion Project site resonated with me as I work to become less judgmental and more open and accepting of others. I use it frequently. It's called the Compassion Exercise. To complete the exercise, focus on a stranger unobtrusively from a distance. Then perform these affirmations:

> "Just like me, this person is seeking happiness in his or her life."
>
> "Just like me, this person is trying to avoid suffering in his or her life."
>
> "Just like me, this person has known sadness, loneliness, and despair."
>
> "Just like me, this person is seeking to fulfill his or her needs."
>
> "Just like me, this person is learning about life."
> (Palmer, 1997)

Although you are instructed to perform all five affirmations, I find I need to do only a few to reframe my thoughts about the person. I go from feeling judgmental about the person to being aware that he or she really is just like me. By practicing this exercise, the hope is that the amount of compassion will increase worldwide.

Another positive affirmation I use—this one by Rudyard Kipling—hangs on my computer at work: "I always prefer to believe the best of everybody, it saves so much trouble" (Kipling, n.d.). It helps me remember that being and becoming a Caritas Coach has tapped into the best of me—something that has always been there but often becomes hidden in the daily grind. It also reminds me that it is up to me to keep these ways of being on display and to help others find them in themselves.

UNITING ALL WAYS OF KNOWING

As part of my studies during the CCEP, I was asked to complete a Caring Science project. For this project I used Carper's patterns of knowing concepts (Carper, 1978; Zander, 2007) and Watson's human Caring Science pedagogy in the development and implementation of a PhD seminar course at the University of Colorado Denver College of Nursing. With a course description and course competencies on hand, I was to develop the course outline, content, readings, assignments, and online engagement activities. This was my first experience developing a new, never-been-taught course.

Doctoral education is personal and reflective. It requires deep engagement and interaction with colleagues and faculty. I felt strongly that enhancing the online course design to encourage student engagement, as well as creativity, would be essential to fostering personal and professional development. I made a list of concepts and activities I thought the course should include to reflect the values of

Caring Science and some of the 10 Caritas Processes. These included the following:

- Starting in-person and synchronous online sessions with a centering activity
- Using check-in and check-out activities in which students intentionally frame how they will engage with the group and identify any issues that may affect their participation, and then affirm how the discussion was valuable to them at the end
- Using SOPHIA (Speak Out, Play Havoc, Imagine Alternatives) to frame their approach to readings and interactions with peers (Wheeler & Chinn, 1991)
- Incorporating multiple and aesthetic ways of knowing into course assignments (Carper, 1978; Zander, 2007)

An instructional designer helped me identify reflective activities in which students could engage. One was the creation of infographics—visual interpretations of course content. Another was "pulse checks." These were brief reflective assessments of progress, epiphanies, or struggles. With each pulse check, I asked students to include a piece of art, a poem, music, an image, or any other form of aesthetic way of knowing that reflected where they were in their learning and thinking. To facilitate personal interaction and engagement, I planned two synchronous online sessions. I also assigned a final paper, which served as a reflective assessment of each student's growth as a Caring Science researcher.

To my delight, students who completed the course actively and creatively engaged in the readings and assignments. Their pulse checks were heartfelt and honest and their aesthetic submissions reflected the depth of their understanding and their personal and professional growth. Ultimately, it was extremely rewarding for me to challenge myself and create something reflective of my new role as a Caritas Coach.

MANIFESTING TRANSPERSONAL CARE

I strive to manifest transpersonal care. A caring moment takes place when I connect on a spirit-to-spirit level with another—beyond personality, physical appearance, behavior, and so on—and I seek to "see" this spirit-filled person (Watson, 2008, p. 82). In my practice, this happens when I authentically listen to the other. I focus on them, not me; make eye contact as appropriate; and set my intention to listen to them. I'm not perfect at this. Sometimes I revert back to my old way of listening, which was to focus on the issue at hand and on finding an answer or solution. But I try not to. Interestingly, I find that when I am successful, the answers still emerge—but in a more thoughtful way.

Another way I manifest transpersonal care is by not getting drawn into the biocidic energy around gossip and judgment. Recall the difficult coworker I mentioned earlier. Many of my colleagues want to talk about her, complain about her communication style, and so on. I try very hard to take the high road and do not encourage this gossip. This means constantly reflecting on my thoughts, actions, and words, and saying what is most helpful to all. I still struggle with this. When colleagues vent I don't always intercede, for fear of seeming rude. However, I recognize that by allowing them to voice their concerns, I am essentially engaging with them—even if I don't say anything negative about the person they are talking about. This is a good example of the ways in which developing the caritas literacies is an ongoing process. My goal is to practice incorporating thoughtful and respectful ways to say, "I am open to your expression of positive and negative feelings, but as a Caritas Coach, I also am committed to finding creative solutions and exploring ways to shift the energy in a more positive direction."

Driving Positivity with Caring Literacy

To have literacy is to have knowledge. To have caring literacy is to weave knowledge, behavior, and intention to make informed conscious decisions. Caring literacy now guides my professional development, as evidenced by what I choose to read and listen to and where I go to learn. Rather than dwell in the negative, I am drawn to the positive.

I strive to find the good in a situation and to hold space for it, and I am learning how to model this approach for others. In my role as educator, I send positive energy to my students as they journey through our doctoral program. When they struggle academically, I engage in deep listening to learn how to best support them.

One of my students, for whom English is her second language, was worried about an upcoming oral presentation. Adding to her stress was the fact that she was repeating the course due to a prior failure. During one practice session, it was clear that she was too nervous to proceed. Instead of urging her to continue, I stopped her, and we talked about strategies she could use to center herself to stay calm and focused. I led her through a brief deep-breathing exercise. As she calmed down, I could see relief on her face. We talked about how she could use this strategy during her presentation. I shared with her how nervous I used to get—and sometimes still do—when speaking in public. This seemed to resonate with her. During her presentation a week later, I saw her use the breathing technique. She was still nervous, but she remained focused, and successfully delivered her presentation.

OPENING ONE'S MIND

A colleague at the college of nursing has a bumper sticker that reads, "Minds are like parachutes. They only function when open." I love this. I live by it and I always have. Caring literacy enhances this attribute in me. I incorporate this openness into my professional development by being willing to experience something new.

Recently, I faced a challenging task: developing and teaching a PhD-level philosophy course related to Caring Science. The course focused on Emmanuel Levinas and Knud Ejler Løgstrup as philosophers whose work was foundational to Watson's Caring Science theory. Never in a million years would I have envisioned myself teaching such a course. Philosophy and theory are not my areas of strength. I spent a good deal of time grappling with this task because I felt so uncomfortable with it.

I said all the typical things to myself. "This will stretch your expertise," I told myself. "It's good to feel uncomfortable and get out of your comfort zone," I said. "It's important to tackle your weaknesses. You will be stronger and smarter." None of these affirmations helped. Then I started thinking about this struggle from a Caritas Coach perspective. This helped me reframe my feelings and self-talk. I told myself this was going to be my first journey of this type. I would start where I was and grow from there. With loving-kindness, I gave myself permission to do the best I could—to focus on progress, not perfection. I honored the process, not just the outcome.

Amazingly, it turned out to be exactly the course I needed to teach and the content I needed to learn. In fact, I thoroughly enjoyed teaching the course. The students and I loved the readings and discussions, and we enjoyed learning together. Aspects of caritas literacy like trusting in myself and being more comfortable with ambiguity were significant in guiding this area of my professional development.

REFLECTING AND ALLOWING

Reflection played a significant role in my Caritas Coach education and continues to have a strong influence on my ongoing development. One way I reflect is through journaling, although this is not yet hard-wired into my routine. I say "yet" because I believe it will be, as one thing I've learned about myself is that I am open to possibilities and new perspectives, and have the ability to do things differently.

Through reflection and self-awareness, I have learned to be patient with myself. This has been extremely important during the past year as I've transitioned into two new roles: faculty in the Caring Science PhD program and a nurse scientist at a children's hospital. Change doesn't happen overnight. Being successful at change requires persistence, hard work, and dedication. Having patience to appreciate the process as it unfolds is part of my new understanding.

I am also trying to have more patience with my family. For some reason, this is not as easy as being patient with myself. I know it will come, however. I have one family member who I don't see often. When we are together, certain aspects of her behavior aggravate me. Naturally, she senses my annoyance. We become distant and tend to avoid each other. Recently, we spent a weekend together. Instead of reacting as I usually do, I tried to refocus my awareness to be intentionally grateful that we had the opportunity to be together, that she is just like me, that we share our love for our family members and each other, and that what I carry in my heart matters. I also focused on our shared love of nature and how it sustains our inner spirit. We both enjoy walks and hikes. I reminded myself we need to do more of these together. We still had our moments, but they were brief and infrequent, and I felt very little of the tension that usually develops between us.

I have taken a deep dive into Caring Science and appreciate all that I am learning and becoming. I strive to be a role model by continuing to practice self-awareness, being quiet, listening, practicing yoga, and taking time for meditation.

FINAL REFLECTIONS

Writing this chapter enabled me to revisit the beautiful uncovering of many of my core beliefs that occurred during my exploration of caritas literacy. Much of what I have recently uncovered had been lying dormant. Now, however, I have language and practices to give voice to my values, beliefs, and actions. I was privileged to study with Dr. Jean Watson, Dr. Sally Gadow, and Dr. Peggy Chinn during my PhD program at the University of Colorado, where the foundation for my worldview took hold. I thank these wonderful women and professors for their important role in my journey as a compassionate and ethical nurse, educator, and Caritas Coach.

REFERENCES

Bradley, A. (2016). International Caritas Consortium Conference keynote address, Boston, MA.

Carper, B. A. (1978). Fundamental patterns of knowing in nursing. *Advances in Nursing Science, 1*(1), 13–23.

Kipling. (n.d.). BrainyQuote.com. Retrieved from https://www.brainyquote.com/quotes/quotes/r/rudyardkip161758.html

Palmer, H. (n.d.). The Avatar Compassion Project. Retrieved from https://theavatarcourse.com/the-compassion-project-eng.html

Palmer, H. (1997). *Resurfacing: Techniques for exploring consciousness*. Altamonte Springs, FL: Star's Edge International.

Watson, J. (1999). *Postmodern nursing and beyond*. London, UK: Churchill Livingstone.

Watson, J. (2008). *Nursing: The philosophy and science of caring* (rev. ed.). Boulder, CO: University Press of Colorado.

Wheeler, C. E., & Chinn, P. L. (1991). *Peace and power: A handbook of feminist process* (3rd ed.). Washington, DC: National League for Nursing Press.

Zander, P. E. (2007). Ways of knowing in nursing: The historical evolution of a concept. *The Journal of Theory Construction & Testing, 11*(1), 7–11.

CARITAS EDUCATION IN CLINICAL SETTINGS

THE CARITAS COACH: AN INSTRUMENT OF HEALING

–Kino Xandro Anuddin, BSN, RN, CNN, HNB-BC, Caritas Coach

Kino describes how his journey to becoming a Caritas Coach empowered him to be more mindful and intentional, and more aware of opportunities to promote caring, love, forgiveness, and mercy for self and other. His ability to stay present, listen with intent, and create open space to simply *be* enables him to care for himself and those around him.

KINO'S CARITAS JOURNEY

When I began training to become a Caritas Coach, I was uncertain of what it meant and what the role required. As a nurse educator, I had assumed that the Caritas Coach Education Program (CCEP) would help me develop knowledge, skills, and abilities to teach and mentor other healthcare colleagues about the application of Caring Science into practice. My time in the CCEP further clarified this understanding. I soon saw the Caritas Coach not as a role to be assumed but as a way of being. More than just learning and teaching the theory of human caring, a Caritas Coach lives the theory, thoughtfully influencing others through sincere words and actions.

SERVING OTHERS

Although caring seems to be a natural social aspect of being human, Jean Watson (2008) suggests that knowledge of caring cannot be taken for granted. Caring Science provides the framework for the development of essential caring literacy on both a personal and a professional level.

Through the study of Caring Science, I have rediscovered what drew me to nursing in the first place: a desire to serve as an instrument of healing. Indeed, in my professional role, my greatest motivation lies in the opportunity to serve others—patients, families, and colleagues. As a nurse, being able to serve people at different phases of their lives brings meaning to my own. Beyond the profession, serving others is simply who I am. It defines my humanity. I feel satisfied when those I serve move toward a better state—whether through healing, growth, learning, improvement, comfort, hope, or what have you. Being a Caritas Coach equips and empowers me to serve effectively and to do so with vigor and meaning.

My knowledge of Caring Science was recently put to the test during an encounter with an adult patient whose kidney disease had progressed to the point that she required dialysis to survive. Her nephrologist had asked me to educate her on her dialysis options.

When I entered her room, I found her distraught. I quickly realized that an attempt to discuss her dialysis options would not be an effective way to serve her. Instead, I placed a chair to her bedside, sat down, touched her hand, and said, "I'm here to listen. Tell me how you feel." The patient explained that although she had tried her best to follow a healthy lifestyle, diabetes and high blood pressure had still damaged her kidneys. She also told me that both her parents had died from kidney disease while receiving hemodialysis. Finally, she shared that she was worried about the burden her treatment might place on her two adult sons. Clearly, the patient was dealing with internal emotional struggles such as anxiety, fear, and guilt. It would have been easy for me to simply reassure the patient that everything would be OK. But I knew that was not what she needed. Instead, I served her by giving her my ears and my time. I think our conversation helped her express her feelings and think through her situation. Afterward, she called her sons, and we scheduled another time to meet so the whole family could be part of the learning and decision-making process.

A Caritas Coach also serves other caregivers and healers, helping them find renewal so they can continue serving their purpose. My goal as a Caritas Coach is to help other nurses reconnect with why they chose nursing as a profession. Nursing is about sharing a journey with others toward healing and comfort. Every nurse has a wonderful opportunity to do just that. Each time they do, it's a beautiful reminder of why they chose to become a nurse. To achieve this, the Caritas Coach takes on different, interconnected roles—educator, leader, friend, colleague, family member—to creatively promote caring, love, forgiveness, compassion, and mercy toward self and other. These are core aspects of being human and humane.

Learning in depth about the 10 Caritas Processes crystallized my understanding of what a Caritas Coach is and what it means to study Caring Science. I realized that the concepts behind these processes mirror the basic principles taught by many religions and philosophies about life, living, and our relationships with others. While each may speak a different "language," they all convey the same truth. In its basic essence, a Caritas Coach inspires others to return to their hearts, find hope, and gather strength. The Caritas Coach empowers others to find the will within themselves to become stronger and more self-sufficient. This is how the Caritas Coach serves others.

Caring Science provides clarity and direction for my role and purpose as a nurse. Understanding my potential to affect others in their healing journey elevates my desire to equip myself with the knowledge, skills, and attitudes needed to be a positive influence. A key aspect of this is mindfulness. Nurses who fail to be mindful of their actions, thoughts, feelings, and choice of words may foster a biocidic relationship or experience with the patient (Halldorsdottir, 1991; Watson, 2008). In contrast, mindful practice of one's thoughts, feelings, words, and actions promotes a safe space for a biogenic healing-growing relationship to flourish while enhancing sensitivity to the state and need of another person.

SEEING FROM THE OTHER'S FRAME OF REFERENCE

As a patient educator, I am often in contact with patients and families to assess learning needs and provide information geared toward health promotion. To achieve this, it is essential that I gain an understanding of each person's needs and the dynamics that exist within each family. In other words, for them to listen to me, I need to listen to them first. To authentically listen—without filter, prejudice, or bias—I must start with myself, by being mindful of my own thoughts and emotions. I must also attempt to see the situation from their frame of reference.

I once cared for an elderly man who spoke only Bengali. As the healthcare team attempted to prepare him for a procedure, the man became very agitated. The team attempted to speak to him using an interpreter, but this proved unproductive, so I called a family member and asked him to come to the hospital to help. While we waited for the family member to arrive, the patient continued speaking loudly in Bengali. I saw fear and alarm in his eyes. I noticed that the situation was also making *me* anxious and nervous. Studying Caring Science has taught me that emotions carry energy that has a way of radiating out and affecting others. The patient's fear was affecting me, and my anxiety was likely affecting him, creating a vicious cycle. I imagined myself in the patient's shoes—being a foreigner in a hospital, unable to communicate with or understand others. That would make me feel unsafe and vulnerable, too! I took a deep breath to calm myself and regain my ground. Then I sat down with the patient and gestured for him to settle down. I attempted to nonverbally communicate to him that I was there to look after him and keep him safe. Finally, he reclined back on his bed and calmed down. He continued to talk to me and I simply listened—although I did not understand his words. After a while, I no longer sensed fear in him. Eventually, the patient's family member arrived. After speaking with the patient in Bengali, the family member explained that the patient thought we were letting him die because he had not been fed for several hours due to the upcoming procedure. It was a clear miscommunication and was eventually resolved.

This experience taught me that healing relationships blossom when trust is present—and that trust grows when a person knows he or she is being heard. It also reminded me that every person comes from a different background, has gone through different experiences, has different values, and holds different perceptions of the world around them. Being receptive, sensitive, and responsive to these differences allows me, as a nurse, to individualize the care I provide in a manner that is most meaningful to the patient.

Nurses will likely be more successful if they engage with the patient and their family as their partner in health; attempt to see things from their "frame of reference" (Watson, 2008, p. 31); and take their expectations, preferences, beliefs, and values into consideration. These are essential steps in developing trusting-caring-healing relationships. As a nurse educator, these same concepts apply when guiding a new associate going through orientation. Any associate who joins a new team comes in with varied experiences, expertise, values, beliefs, and preferred methods of learning. Honoring these differences is important—not just for the new team member, but for the whole team. This involves guiding existing staff in integrating their new colleague into the culture.

LISTENING WITH INTENT

I believe I possess a strong capacity to hold space for others by listening. One of my mentors validated this when she described how she sees me affect others—the way I convey my presence by listening with intent. For example, I tend not to interrupt others when they speak. I try to simply listen rather than mentally formulating my next response. This may sound like nothing more than just good manners, but listening in this way makes others feel they are valuable, important, and worthy of my time.

In the poem "Desiderata," Max Ehrmann (1948) writes, "... listen to others, even to the dull and the ignorant; they too have their story." When people share their story with me, I take it as an indication of their trust. I can best honor that trust by listening. I can also gain a deeper understanding of their values, beliefs, and perceptions. As a nurse, helping others find sense and meaning in their own story is a valuable way to guide them toward a path of healing. Jean Watson (2008) explains that allowing others to freely express their thoughts and feelings without judgment is a healing act in itself. It facilitates spirit-to-spirit connection, creating a two-way nurse-patient transpersonal caring-healing experience.

The project I completed as part of the CCEP involved the creation of mandalas by patients receiving hemodialysis treatment. Creating mandalas has long been used as a way to encourage self-reflection, self-expression, insight, and healing (Dossey & Keegan, 2016). As part of the mandala project, I engaged the dialysis staff in creating a safe and trusting space for patients to color pre-printed mandalas during their 3 to 4 hours of dialysis treatment. The goal of the activity was two-fold. First, to provide an opportunity for patients to reflect on their thoughts, emotions, or personal goals, and to creatively express those through their mandalas. Second, to engage the staff in helping patients find meaning in their mandalas by practicing active listening and curiosity, not judgment. Although the activity itself may seem simple, it provided a beautiful opportunity for our patients and staff to know each other on a different level.

One elderly patient created a very colorful floral mandala with each petal representing one of her grandchildren. This revealed to the nurse caring for the patient the value of her grandchildren. The nurse took the initiative to make a phone call to give the patient a chance to speak with some of her grandchildren that day. "I was so glad I was able to do that for her," the nurse later told me. "Her smile spoke volumes." This is a wonderful example of a transpersonal moment with a heartfelt connection made between the nurse and patient.

Taking time to slow down and just *be* so you can listen has its own rewards. It is quite normal to feel pressured by the need to complete daily tasks. I often catch myself rushing to get things done. But grounding myself in the moment and releasing the ties that pull my attention to other things enable me to intentionally be present for others. I do this in simple ways, such as pausing and taking a deep breath before entering a patient's room and practicing heart-focused breathing as I walk to my next meeting. Acknowledging that all my choices, actions, and words can influence how a situation unfolds and how they can affect another person—not only in the immediate moment but also in moments after—raises my sense of responsibility to be mindful of my own presence.

CARING LITERACY

One premise of Caring Science is that caring literacy cannot be assumed (Watson, 2008). Although it is natural for people to care, caring literacy requires continuous self-awareness and self-growth and the cultivation of emotional heart intelligence, caring consciousness, and intentionality to effectively guide others in their healing journey. To convey authentic presence within the caring-healing relationship, ongoing attention to different ways of doing and being is also required.

Caring literacies are caring attributes translated into actions. Therefore, they represent the essential knowledge, skills, and ways of being to manifest caring. Just like learning a new skill or language, cultivating caring literacy requires patience and purposeful practice. Every situation or encounter is a potential opportunity to practice caring literacy. Therefore, it is important to carefully consider how each situation can serve as an effective teaching-learning moment in developing one's own caring literacy.

For me, growing professionally as a nurse, educator, and leader requires self-direction and motivation. Aligning that growth with Caring Science provides a clear definition of who I am to be—and become—as a nurse, educator, and leader. An effective starting point for me is examining how I integrate the 10 Caritas Processes in my professional practice. I find that I can apply these processes in multiple ways depending on what each situation requires. As a caritas practitioner, it is up to me to develop the necessary sensitivity, intuition, and creativity to respond to a particular situation with care and compassion. This requires an ability to "read the field" (Watson, 2008, p. 25) and is nurtured by being present in the moment.

Reading the field also comes into play in my role as a provider of learning resources for the nursing staff in my hospital. In addition to identifying learning needs by assessing gaps in the standards of practice and reviewing new or high-risk procedures that require competency to ensure safe practice, I remain open to the subjective signs that tell me whether a learner is engaged in the learning process or if certain barriers exist. In other words, I read the field. Paying attention to these subtle signs enables me to adjust my teaching strategy to better connect with the learner and more effectively meet learning goals.

Caring Science acknowledges that there are multiple ways of knowing (Zander, 2007). One can draw truth, insight, creativity, and inspiration by integrating the various ways of knowing into practice. Embracing all ways of knowing supports open-mindedness, curiosity, and a nonjudgmental attitude toward others.

FINDING PURPOSE

I have made a personal and ethical commitment to look after my own well-being physically, mentally, emotionally, and spiritually. It is a personal commitment because I do it for my own good. Consciously performing self-care helps me promote a healthy body, mind, and spirit. It also helps me feel good about myself, maintain confidence, and enjoy a good quality of life. It is an ethical responsibility because a healthy me contributes to a healthy community. As a nurse, being healthy means I am best able to perform my role in caring, helping, and healing others. This role requires more than just an able body. It also requires a mind and heart capable of connecting and responding to others with love and compassion.

I consider myself an introvert. I'm introspective. It is natural for me to look inward before looking outward. I process stimuli by internalizing. Although I know every person I encounter and every situation I experience are opportunities for learning, these lessons can easily pass right by without notice if I do not take time to reflect on them. To do this, I begin each day by setting an intention of being aware of things to be grateful for throughout the day. Then, at the end of the day, as I drive home from work or before I retire for sleep, I recall situations and encounters from the day. I reflect on my actions, words, responses, thoughts, and feelings during these moments and try to learn from them. I ask myself, what went well? What could have gone differently? How have I affected others? I know I can't change what has already happened, but I can always do something better the next time around.

Writing down my thoughts and experiences in a journal has also been helpful in exploring my own consciousness. Journaling helps me identify specific behaviors or patterns and find meaning in them. Journaling also helps me see how my thinking, personality, and very consciousness evolve over time. I have been journaling for only 2 years, but whenever I go back and read what I've written, I gain insight into my own growth as a person.

Daily life can be overwhelming. Everything is continuously moving and changing. It's easy to feel mentally and emotionally exhausted, lost in what is (or what we think should be) happening. In a fast-paced environment—not to mention a society that seemingly values productivity above all else—being still, thinking, and reflecting can feel like an inefficient use of time. But the continuous buildup of stress adversely affects one's productivity and one's ability to focus and be present with others. It also affects one's personal health and well-being. Allowing myself space to be still in silence is an essential component of my self-care. In silence I hear best, and in stillness I see movement. I must allow myself that space so I can understand myself more clearly.

Practicing self-reflection through heart-focused breathing, journaling, creative arts, and introspective meditation helps me become self-aware. It is through this awareness that I can seek ways to attend to my needs and practice self-care. It is also from this awareness that I gain sensitivity and insight to recognize what a patient, family member, or colleague may need and respond accordingly.

FINAL REFLECTIONS

My evolving journey of being and becoming a Caritas Coach continuously deepens my understanding of my role and purpose as a nurse and as a person. As a Caritas Coach, I am endlessly motivated to serve by guiding others in finding meaning in their work and in their relationships with others. Finding my own life purpose and meaning requires self-reflection. In this way, I gain awareness of the influence of my thoughts, feelings, words, and actions on others and myself. From this awareness, I am able to develop the sensitivity required to appropriately respond to the needs of others and to continually be present with them in the moment.

As a Caritas Coach, I am dedicated to constant personal and professional development. This is a lifelong process. Maintaining openness to multiple ways of knowing helps me attain open-mindedness, curiosity, and creativity for problem-solving and decision-making.

Acknowledging that every situation offers opportunities to learn, to practice caring literacy, and to teach others about caring literacy and the 10 Caritas Processes enables me to stay grounded, be present in each moment, and see my path as a healer with more clarity.

REFERENCES

Dossey, B. M., & Keegan, L. (2016). *Holistic nursing: A handbook for practice* (7th ed.). Burlington, MA: Jones & Bartlett Learning.

Ehrmann, M. (1948). Desiderata. *The poems of Max Ehrmann.* (B. Ehrmann, Ed.). Boston, MA: Bruce Humphries, Inc. Retrieved from https://en.wikipedia.org/wiki/Desiderata#cite_note-platt-1

Halldorsdottir, S. (1991). *Five basic modes of being with another.* In D. A. Gaut and M. Leininger (Eds.), *Caring: The compassionate healer.* New York, NY: National League for Nursing.

Watson, J. (2008). *Nursing: The philosophy and science of caring* (rev. ed.). Boulder, CO: University Press of Colorado.

Zander, P. E. (2007). Ways of knowing in nursing: The historical evolution of a concept. *Journal of Theory Construction & Testing, 11*(1), 7–11.

LIVING CARITAS

–CHRISTINE GRIFFIN, MS, RN, CPN,
CARITAS COACH, MASTER HEARTMATH TRAINER

By sharing stories about caring for children, Chris demonstrates how Caring Science guides her to discover the uniqueness of each child and family. As she reflects on each story, Chris shares her own inner journey toward deeper knowing and ultimate wisdom. Importantly, Chris openly explores where she falls short and how she reflects on these experiences through the lens of Caring Science so that she can grow as a Caritas Coach and humanitarian.

CHRIS'S CARITAS JOURNEY

What does it mean to be and become a Caritas Coach? For me, it means everything. The philosophy and science of caring not only helps me sustain my nursing practice, it enables me to flourish within the complexities of caring for others.

Like many nurses, I entered a healthcare profession because I wanted to make a difference and help others heal. My childhood heroes were people who were selfless helpers. I specifically wanted to care for children in a hospital setting. This is where I knew I could make the most difference.

Even before my nursing practice had a foundation of Caring Science, I was able to care. In fact, I cared profoundly for my patients and their families. I was considered a good bedside nurse. I always put each patient's needs before my own. Indeed, I cared for the patient's whole family and made sure all their needs were met. I felt there was no limit to what I could do to help someone else. This is what nurses do, right? Our endless supply of care is the most important and fulfilling part of our job. Unfortunately, this was not the whole story. I began to feel worn down. My body began to hurt. I was in emotional pain. I had nothing left to give my husband and children because I had already given everything I had to others. I justified this by telling myself it was part of the job. This is what I had signed up for. I just needed to work through it and keep giving.

For a while, making a difference—even a small one—was enough to sustain me. Each night I told myself I had helped someone that day. That was what mattered. Then something happened. One of my primary patients—someone I cared deeply about—passed away. She was only 3 years old. She literally died in my arms. I broke. I gave up on caring. I built walls to protect what little bit of myself was left. As I did, I became very aware that I was no longer the type of nurse I wanted to be. I was no longer inspired. I was no longer caring. This was even more painful.

By some small miracle, I met Dr. Jean Watson. Watson and the Caritas Coach Education Program (CCEP) put me on a path that focused not on suffering but on peace. It was a path of reflection, not shame; of hope, not despair. I began to remember my purpose on Earth. Most importantly, I learned a structure and language that enabled me to care deeply for others while flourishing in my own self-awareness and self-care.

The CCEP helped me understand that being selfless doesn't mean you value yourself less. It is more about learning to focus on your own truth in relation to another. We assess our own worth and authentic self by how it connects to another. In studying Caring Science, we learn that in transpersonal relationships, both people matter. A foundation of caring literacy enables the nurse to be authentically present with each patient and clear on the importance of self-care. We see our own humanity in what the other experiences. Therefore, by caring for them, we actually care for ourselves. We walk toward wholeness so we can wholly care for another. I wasn't whole before (although I was able to fake it really well). My patients received broken care from a broken soul.

Thanks to the CCEP, I am back to being the nurse I always dreamed of being. I have reconnected with my passion for caring and have found an endless source of energy to sustain it. I know the difference I can make as a healthcare provider and the simple steps I can perform to take care of myself and others in the same moment. The CCEP opened my eyes and heart. I gained a new depth of understanding of what it means to be a nurse.

It has also opened space for me to help other nurses use these tools to be and become all they can be as caregivers—to walk toward their own wholeness as they learn to walk others toward theirs, and to see their own humanity as they look for it in others. This is critical. To survive as a caring profession, nursing must begin to teach the skills needed for both the patient *and* the nurse to move toward wholeness. As Watson reminds us, "A caring attitude is not transmitted from generation to generation by genes. It is transmitted by the culture of society. The culture of nursing, in this instance the discipline and profession of nursing has a vital social scientific role in advancing, sustaining and preserving human caring as a way of fulfilling its mission to society and broader humanity" (Watson, 2008, p. 18).

I recognize myself when I see nurses who are burned out or feel the effects of compassion fatigue. Watson tells us, "We learn from one another how to be more human by identifying ourselves with others and finding their dilemmas in ourselves. We learn to recognize ourselves in others" (Watson, 2008, p. 5). By being more mindful of my own suffering, I am more open to my colleagues. Watson says, "By being sensitive to our own presence and caritas consciousness, not only are we able to offer and enable another to access his or her own belief systems of faith-hope for the person healing, but we may be the one who makes the difference between hope and despair in a given moment" (Watson, 2008, p. 62). As a caritas nurse, I have the tools and knowledge to return hope to the hopeless nurse. Together we can raise our levels of consciousness to help each other heal as we create space for our patients and families to heal.

Throughout this journey, I have experienced so many meaningful interactions and lessons. Much of what I have learned has come from reflections on my nursing practices. In my journey as a nurse—and of being and becoming a caritas nurse—there are countless examples of how my thinking and practice have shifted. I have shared some here to illustrate how Caring Science has shaped me into the nurse and person I am today.

FREEING MYSELF OF MY EGO

Even in moments where caring is the intention, our fear, self-doubt, and ego can get in the way. I will never forget the lesson one patient taught me about how my own needs—even when they come from a good place—block true presence and inhibit connection and healing.

One of the most meaningful experiences for me when I am at work is when I connect with a pediatric patient. I try hard to help the kids in my care feel like they are not in the hospital—to help them forget they're being poked and prodded and are hooked up to machines and IVs. My favorite way to do this is through age-appropriate humor. I'll do anything to make them laugh. I tell teenagers I am afraid of blood and ask if it is OK if I close my eyes while I start their IVs. Or I put something silly on my head and "sneeze," catapulting the item into a toddler's lap. They can't help but laugh. Their bodies relax, and everyone in the room just breathes easier. I want to remind these kids and their families that their diagnosis is just a word. Nothing more. It need not define their every moment. In fact, recognizing that kids still need to be kids even when they are sick helps the entire family deal better with what they must face.

Enter Guy. Guy was a 16-year-old patient who functioned at a lower developmental and cognitive level than other teenagers his age. He was very sick. He had undergone several surgeries. He could not tolerate food. He had tubes everywhere. Guy communicated only with his family, in their Native American language. With nurses and other staff Guy simply moaned and grunted. When he needed something, he would point and moan. When he was mad at you, he would grunt and point to the door in the hopes that you would leave.

As someone who was called into Guy's room to administer a lot of pokes and procedures, I got a lot of grunts from Guy. In his mind, I was someone who hurt him. Even if I was just checking on the family, the minute I came into the room, Guy would give me a mean look (although he refused to make eye contact) and point to the door. My ego did not like this. Remember, I was a nurse who made everything better! I made it my mission to win Guy over—to help him see what a great nurse I was. Every day I went to his bedside and brought him gifts—bribes, really. I made jokes—I'd even get his family laughing—but Guy would just grunt and point at the door. Nothing worked. Worse, every time I came in the room, Guy became stressed and angry.

I finally took a hard look at myself. I realized I was doing all of this for me—for my bruised ego—not for Guy. In trying to win him over, I was only causing him more frustration and pain. This is not something a caritas nurse does. We can't force caring moments, no matter how badly we want to. So I decided to back off. I stopped going to Guy's bedside unless I needed to. In his room, I always gave him a quick smile, but then I gave him space as I addressed his family. I also built a trusting relationship with Guy's mom. I went out of my way to make her comfortable. Guy seemed to like this. He loved his mom very much. Eventually Guy stopped grunting when I was in the room. He no longer stiffened up at the sight of me. In time, I was able to quietly approach Guy and put my hand on his shoulder. I would tell him I was happy to see him and that I hoped he'd had a good day. He still refused to make eye contact but he seemed to understand that I was not the enemy. This didn't happen overnight. Guy was with us for more than 3 months.

One night, after Guy had undergone yet another surgery and had even more tubes protruding from his body, another nurse asked me to hang his antibiotic. I went into the room and set it up without a word. Guy's mom had gone to dinner so Guy was alone watching *The Jungle Book*. Two main characters, Mowgli and Baloo the Bear, began singing "Bare Necessities," and I quietly sang along. Guy looked up at me and smiled. He approved that I knew the song. When I started to leave, Guy did something I will never forget: He reached for my hand. Then, still holding my hand, he pointed to the chair to indicate that he wanted me to sit down. I sat down. He squeezed my hand and smiled at me, and we watched the movie together in silence. He never let go, even when I had to fight back some tears. He just held my hand. In doing so, he gave me the most amazing gift possible—without evening knowing it.

I will never forget that moment. It changed how I approach every situation: without my ego and just with my heart. By creating healing space for another, we create healing space for ourselves. We are all connected. I know that Guy was sent to me as a lesson, and I am so grateful for my time with him. Whenever my ego gets in the way, I picture Guy's face when he reached for my hand and changed my heart. This is what a caritas nurse does. We meet others at their level, not ours—for their needs, not ours—to hold them in their humanity until they can hold themselves.

Becoming the Environment

For nurses in a hospital setting, the pace is unrelenting. But it is often our patients who pay the real price for this. Even as patients plumb the depths of suffering and illness, the one person who can offer hope and healing is instead focused on ticking boxes on a to-do list—a list that often overlooks what the patient truly needs to heal. As a caritas nurse, I know the difference I can make by stepping away from this "just get things done" approach. By being still, at right relation first with myself and then with others, I can give the gift of presence. I am not simply in an environment with another; for better or worse, according to Watson, "the nurse is the environment" (Watson, 2008, p. 26). This lesson became clear to me in the care of one of my young patients.

I work on the pulmonary unit in my hospital. We take care of the trach and vent population. These are usually children who are less than a year old and cannot breathe on their own. The vent keeps them alive in the hopes that one day they will no longer need its support to breathe. These children suffer endless respiratory treatments to help keep their lungs open. They are constantly suctioned and repositioned. It's not easy for them. The hardest part is that they endure all this without a voice. They cannot tell us if we are meeting their needs. In fact, they cannot make any noise at all—not even when they cry. (Interestingly, I believe I have had my most meaningful caring moments with the patients who cannot tell you what they are thinking!)

One of my vent patients was a little boy named Josiah. At first I was so nervous about the machinery attached to him that it was easy to forget he was even there. But as I grew more comfortable, I began noticing subtle changes in him anytime I was authentically present—when I took time to meet his physical, emotional, and spiritual needs. I gave him long baths. At bedtime, I sang to him. He always fell asleep much faster for me than for anyone else.

I quickly learned that Josiah loved to watch *Mickey Mouse Clubhouse* on TV. I began arranging my day with my other patients so I could sit with Josiah and we could watch the show together. As I held him, we would sing (although Josiah's singing was silent) and clap hands, and he would smile and laugh his silent laugh. Then I started singing one of the songs anytime I came into his room so he would know it was me who was coming. Each time I sang that song and entered his room, the environment changed. Josiah would turn and smile at me. We both understood that this was our time together. (Interestingly, this practice also became a way for me to center myself. When I sang the "Hot Dog Dance" song, I knew I was going to be with Josiah, and I would intentionally release all of my stress to be present just for him.) I brought him clothes so he could wear something other than hospital gowns.

I believe this is what transpersonal practice is all about: meeting the needs of the other by just being present, centered, and authentic. By creating an environment. Josiah knew I cared about him. He knew he could trust me. When I was with him he knew he was safe and loved. In turn, I knew I was meeting his needs. He could not tell me but he showed me. He showed me with his body language and his smile. He showed me with his relaxed muscles and his calmness. Even his vital signs reflected his happy and content state.

When Josiah left the hospital to go home, I gave him a Mickey Mouse watch on a chain. I told his mom that the time I spent with him was more like play than work, and that whenever I heard our song I would think of our special time together. Josiah was the one who received a gift that day. But when I am authentically present with patients, the gifts I receive from them far outweigh any gifts they receive from me.

In my morning huddles with nurses I often challenge them to change a patient's environment for the better. This might be something as simple as telling the patient, "I am grateful that I am your nurse today." This simple act can change the entire mood of the room. In the afternoon, I check back with my nurses and we celebrate the creative ways they found to change the patient's environment. I plan to continue with this practice. We also help our nurses stay centered as they administer care to patients by posting a sign labeled "Pause to Care" outside each patient's room. It serves as a reminder to center and breathe before entering a patient's environment. I want to go on looking for ways to inspire others to be truly present and centered so they can develop real transpersonal relationships with their patients and the patients' families.

IN THE MOMENT WE ARE EQUAL

Transpersonal caring is the gold standard for care between two people. It means that one can see oneself in the other and that we both matter. It means that in this moment we are equal. Indeed, it is only when one sees the other as an equal that compassion can occur. Pema Chödrön writes, "Compassion is not a relationship between the healer and the wounded. It's a relationship between equals. Only when we know our own darkness well can we be present with the darkness of others. Compassion becomes real when we recognize our shared humanity" (2008, p. 74).

I used to think caring moments just happened naturally. If I was a good nurse, every patient would know my heart. When this did not happen, I believed it was because I failed. But now that I have a foundation in Caring Science I know that these moments do not always just happen. They come from being in right relation with myself first so I can then be in right relation with others. I must be able to center and see the spirit-filled person behind the diagnosis, and the patient must be willing to be vulnerable and receive care. As Watson writes, "Caring is such a vulnerable place; first because we come face-to-face with our own humanity and ourselves. In this place, we realize that one person's level of humanity reflects back on the other...We are remembering we are touching the life force, the very soul of another person, hence ourselves" (Watson, 2005, p. 61). Indeed, Watson reminds us over and over that when we understand the connectedness and oneness of all humanity, cruelty to another becomes intolerable (Watson, 2005; Watson, 2008). We see another's body and soul as our own body and soul and we treat both with a new kind of reverence and care.

Being in this space with another human is the biggest gift we offer to humanity. I cannot think of a better way to describe this than to share a story about a little girl who brought out the best and worst in me both as a person and as a nurse. Her diagnosis brought me fear but her heart taught me about humility and grace. Her name was Abbi. Abbi had epidermolysis bullosa (EB). EB is a complicated diagnosis. It's often referred to as "the worst disease you have never heard of." Children with EB have extremely fragile skin that blisters and tears from minor friction. They are often covered in bandages. They endure a life of infection and pain and often lose their battle with the disease at a very young age. What follows are my reflections about my journey with Abbi from the moment I met her to the time I had to say goodbye.

You are my....

Your disease was pure evil. I don't like that word but it is the only way I can describe how awful it was. Your fragile body came apart at the skin. Where was the glue that others have? Why did my skin stay on while yours fell off? What was God thinking?

You are my....

You smiled. You laughed. You took challenges in stride like only an old soul can—one who understands that life isn't fair but the only choice is to fight and live and teach.

When I met you I was scared. I didn't want to go in the room. I didn't want to touch you. I didn't want to be your nurse because I would have to see your pain. I might have to come to terms with not being able to help you. I might suffer. I might cry.

We connected. I pushed my fear away and led with my heart. *She is just a child*, I told myself. *Get her to laugh. Help her play. Help her forget. If she forgets then so can you. Forget the limitations. Forget the prognosis.*

Just forget.

You needed to change your dressings. No, not that! I had heard the screams.

You needed to take a bath with bleach. Please God don't make me be there. The fear resurfaced.

No, I thought. *Lead with your heart. Be present. Bring love with you.* "Let's play," I said. "I promise this will be the best bath you have ever had." You got in the bath lickety-split. Oh, the pain from the bleach on those open sores must have been unbearable. "Here's a syringe," I said. "Shoot water at me!" Yes, the water with the bleach, with the skin, with the blood. *Squirt.* Was that a smile? *Squirt.* Was that a laugh? I was soaked. I didn't care. I didn't feel it. You and I splashed and squirted. We spilled water everywhere. People came to check on us. "Are you OK?" they asked. Yes. We were OK.

You were done bathing but you didn't want to stop. *The pain has to be there*, I thought. A water fight can't remove the facts of bleach and open wounds. But you didn't care. The pain was normal for you. Playing during the pain, however—*that* was a new experience. *Please don't let it end*, I thought. *For either of us.*

You are my...

We fought to spend time together. Other nurses, other patients—they didn't matter. You and I needed each other. You got to laugh at me. I got to feel human. I made a difference when I was your nurse.

You called for me on the call light. "Abbi," I said. "I have other patients. Do you need me?"

"No," you replied. "I just want you to come. When can you come?"

The answer was always "Now." I couldn't take away your disease. I usually couldn't take away the pain. I could give you only three things: my heart, my presence, and my care. Care. That's what I gave you. I cared for you. I cared about you. I cared.

You are my...

I saw you several times a year—more when you were sick. You told me stories of your life. Horses. Family. Your disease and medications. Fun combined with pain. Always the pain. You taught me something new each time I saw you. You were vulnerable with me. You knew you could cry. You knew you could be grumpy. I shouldered your anger when it spilled over. I didn't mind. I was grateful you trusted me with every emotion. You couldn't scare me anymore. I was your nurse. I was meant to be that. We were placed on each other's path and you became part of my story.

You are my...

You were on your death bed. You were 9 years old. Still you fought. "I don't want to go to heaven without you, Mommy," you said. Your mother was not ready. I was not ready. You were not ready. *Damn it.* I thought. *Can't she at least choose when she is ready?* Unfair. Unjust. Evil disease.

I went to you—not alone, with a fellow nurse. Nurses can't do this part alone. It was near the end. You were there in body—though you were still. Unmoving. But your mind—your soul—was somewhere else. I prayed it was somewhere safe—away from here, away from the waiting, from all these people staring at you. People who didn't know what to do with their sadness, who were scared fragile, whose emotions wouldn't help anyone. People like me.

I talked to you. I thanked you. I lied and said it was
OK. I lied and said that your mom would be OK.
She will be—but not for a long time. I told you how
you changed me to my core. I wasn't sure you could
hear me. I wasn't sure I wanted you to hear me. My
words were more for me—my closure, my needs, my
suffering.

You were imprinted on my heart. Sometimes I
wondered if there was a spot on your heart for me. I
got my answer that day—that last time we touched
hands. You told me everything I needed to know
without saying a word. Lying there in your pain
medication–induced slumber, your eyes were open.
I reminded you that I hated it when you slept with
your eyes open. You always freaked me out with
that trick.

And you, Abbi, you closed your eyes for me.

In this way, you told me you cared for me. You told
me that this journey was one we took together—that
even now, at the end, we mattered to each other. Just
by closing your eyes you banished my fears and my
feelings of failure.

I could not always take away your pain. I could not
always make you laugh. I could not always make
you forget your prognosis or give you hope for tomorrow. But I did connect with you. I did find a way
into your heart. We did reach each other—a nurse
and her special patient.

You are my...

My patient, my friend, my hero, my heart.

I am still processing this loss, looking at it from new ways of knowing and becoming. Watson reminds us that we cannot skip the painful parts of life. We must walk through joy *and* suffering to find meaning and purpose. "It seems we learn through the deeply personal encounters with suffering that we cannot go around life, we have to go through the experience in order to not only survive but to thrive, to sustain a sense of hope for continued existence, living" (Watson, 2005, p. 134). Watson teaches us that we can move toward joy *while pain is present*. Doing this for ourselves is one thing. Being able to help others in this process is a true gift.

PULLING OTHERS UP

Caritas calls on us to pull from our deepest humanity to hold others up until they can do it for themselves. I was proud to be among a group of nurses who did this for one family in distress. This family belonged to a little girl named Jenny.

Jenny had an anorexia brain injury at home. EMTs had revived Jenny at the scene, but she had been neurologically devastated. Jenny's family was grief-stricken. They were angry, terrified, and consumed with guilt. They were not ready to let go of their little girl—not when she was so broken. Even though Jenny's doctors told them Jenny would never get better, they pushed the doctors to place Jenny on a ventilator. When Jenny contracted an infection that went out of control, her family insisted on fighting it—even asking for extreme measures including amputation.

Jenny received this care at another facility. Then she was transferred to the facility where I worked. When she arrived on my unit, she was in poor condition. She was what we call "riding the ventilator," meaning she did not take any spontaneous breaths on her own. She had bed sores on several areas of her body. Her skin was so fragile that even a simple touch tore at her skin. She rarely opened her eyes. When she did she would cry.

This was the patient we started with—but it was not the end of the story. You see, I work on a unit filled with caritas nurses—nurses who look for and therefore find humanity in every situation, who look for connections and therefore make them, who look for the person behind the diagnosis. They don't ask *if* they can care. They ask what is the best way to care for this patient in this moment.

We knew Jenny would not recover from her brain injury. We could not hope for the miracle of a full recovery. So we asked ourselves what we *could* hope for. The answers were clear. First, we could hope to support the family. Second, we could hope to manage Jenny's pain. And third, we could hope Jenny would feel love. Surprisingly, we could realize all three of these hopes with one simple approach: treating Jenny like we would if we knew she would get better. That meant believing in possibilities, ignoring limitations, expecting the miracle, and never looking back. So that is what we did.

We took care of her skin, and her bedsores healed. Her amputation site healed, and eventually we were able to remove the bandage. We administered medicine and treatments to make her stronger. More importantly, we talked to her, sang to her, and held her. We bathed her and dressed her and did her hair, as though each day was the day she would go home to play with her brothers and sisters. Slowly she calmed more easily and cried less. She began to heal in all the ways her broken body could.

As for her family, we took care of them, too—although they were not always easy to deal with. So consumed by anger and guilt and grief, they rarely visited Jenny. It was too painful. And when they did, they often told us how poorly we were caring for their daughter. But we kept caring. When they gave us anger, we gave them compassion. When they gave us frustration, we showed empathy.

Ever so slowly, as Jenny began to look better, her mother started to visit more often. She started to bring in more outfits for Jenny and to pick out what she wanted Jenny to wear the next day. She gave suggestions on hairstyles. She told us Jenny's favorite songs and TV programs so we could play them for Jenny when she wasn't here.

She brought more family members to visit Jenny—including Jenny's siblings. She started to hold Jenny—to talk to her—like she saw us do.

More significantly, Jenny's mother started to come to terms with the limitations of her daughter's diagnosis. She began to let go of a future with her daughter and to take things moment to moment. Eventually, she began to ask us what we thought about end of life for Jenny. What would it look like? Would Jenny suffer? Was there any chance for a recovery? Would Jenny think we gave up on her? These were hard questions. There were no simple answers. But there were *caring* answers, and those were the answers we gave. Answers like, "We are here for you." "We are with you." We also asked Jenny's mother one question of our own: What do you want for your daughter? At first, the answer was, "I want her back." Then it changed to, "I want her to not suffer anymore." And finally it became, "I want her to be at peace." It was then that Jenny's family had the strength to make the best decision she could for Jenny: to remove her from the ventilator.

Jenny did not receive the miracle of recovery. But she did receive the miracle of care. And her family received the miracle of getting to see their daughter whole again before she passed on. They did not have to let go of her while she was broken. She was their little girl with possibilities and potential, and they will always see her that way. Ram Dass has said, "We're all just walking each other home" (n.d.). Jenny's nurses did that. We did that. While holding the hands of Jenny's family, we walked Jenny home.

WALKING TOWARD AUTHENTIC BEING

It is only through self-awareness—through reflection and stillness—that I can walk toward my own authentic being. The experiences on which I reflect are not always positive, however. I have seen real pain in my experiences caring for others—pain endured by my patients and their families and my own pain due to my limitations in a given moment.

I carry with me the times I did not stay present or I put my own needs over those of another. Indeed, I remember more of my momentary lapses than my moments of caring. One painful moment involved a young patient on end-of-life care to whom I was assigned and who was expected to pass away during my shift. This was not an unusual assignment for me.

I was viewed as someone who could handle difficult situations so I was frequently assigned some of the most difficult care environments. But I was faking it. I appeared to have it all together, but the truth was I was well on my way to burning out.

I did not know if I had it in me to go through this experience with another child and family. But before I could protest, the patient's monitor sounded. I hurried to his room to see what was happening. When I entered, the physician was at the boy's bedside along with his parents. "We decided to turn off the oxygen so this is not prolonged," the physician said. Then he left the room. The phrase "intimate strangers" describes when you share a very sacred moment with someone without really knowing them. This was exactly that. I did not know the patient's full name or his exact age. Nor did I know his mom's or dad's name. Yet there I was with them during a tragic and life-changing moment.

The patient did not die right away. He continued to breathe on his own for several more hours. He did not appear to be suffering. I never saw him awake. I never saw him open his eyes. He lay still, his grieving parents on either side of him. I cared for him and his parents until he passed and stayed with them until they were ready to say their final goodbyes. I held his mom as she cried. His dad was harder to comfort. He just had a distant look on his face. We didn't talk much. The only thing I could offer him was a hand on his shoulder. After they thanked me several times, they left the hospital. As for me, I prepared the boy's body, wheeled him down to our morgue, and returned to my unit for my next assignment.

Here's the part I regret: the dread I felt during those hours in that room. I did not want to be there. I wanted someone else to come in and take over. I wanted to run away. I wanted to cry. I wanted to scream. I wanted to break down and crawl in a corner. Of course, none of these responses were allowed. So instead I just told myself I wanted it to be over. I needed it to be over. I remember saying in my mind, over and over, "Fly to Jesus. Fly to Jesus. Fly to Jesus. Please just fly to Jesus." I was very weak in this moment—almost broken. This is not how a caregiver is supposed to feel. I was not fully present for three people who needed me then more than ever. But I couldn't help it.

I never saw or heard from them again. I pray I came across to them as present and caring. I will never know what their experience was or if they even remember me. But whether they remember me or not, I will never forget them. My heart still aches for them—so much so that if someone asked me if I could go back in time for a do-over, this would be at the top of my list. If I could do things over, I would show up. I would be kinder. More present. Less selfish. I would just be in the moment and appreciate the honor of being chosen to share an experience with intimate strangers.

This moment in time is forever embedded in my heart. But as I look for the lesson, I must also look for the compassion I need to forgive myself and heal. I'm still working on that.

THE IMPORTANCE OF HOPE

I see levels of consciousness as rungs on a ladder. Fear, hatred, and ego are the lowest rungs. As such, they are easily accessible. Reaching them does not involve much personal risk. The higher rungs—compassion, self-awareness, love, and hope—are much harder to reach. For many, the climb is too risky. They don't even try. Reaching these rungs requires motivation, persistence, and the courage to keep climbing. But much like climbing a ladder can reveal a spectacular view, reaching these higher levels of consciousness can help us to see the beauty in our lives and world. It is worth the climb.

I believe the highest level of consciousness a nurse offers his or her patients is hope. Hope is not a belief. It is an action—seeing something that may not exist yet and wholeheartedly pursuing it. In healthcare, however, hope is often denied. This is because our current medical model demands that providers cure rather than heal—that they relieve a symptom rather than restore wholeness. In contrast, caritas asks us to honor the awe, wonder, beauty, mystery, and miracles of humankind (Watson, 2008). To be open to the spiritual—to the mysteries and unknowns that allow miracles to occur. In short, to not just let hope exist, but to allow it to flourish.

For me, the importance of hope is best illustrated by an experience I had with a family whose son came into this world broken. The boy's parents were not from this country and held different cultural beliefs. They had been convinced that by bringing their son to our modern hospital, he would be cured. When this did not happen—when they lost hope their son would ever be "normal"—they lashed out. Each step of the boy's care brought anger and accusations. The boy's father was particularly angry. He yelled at us constantly. "I could write a book!" he'd say before launching into all the ways we were failing him and his son. He simply did not believe we cared for him or his son. It was a hostile environment to say the least.

We could have matched anger with anger, threats with consequences. Instead, we used all 10 Caritas Processes—from loving-kindness, to being open to miracles, to seeing hope in the midst of despair, to creating space for negative and positive emotions—to help this man and his family. I placed special emphasis on creating a space where he was safe to express both positive and negative emotions. Toward the end of the stay, when he'd start on a new "I could write a book" rant, I would reply that *my* chapter in this book was all about hope—not for the perfect son he imagined, but for the son who had been perfectly made for his love.

Eventually, the boy's father did begin to believe I was someone he could count on. When they left he thanked me. He even gave me a hug! And although he could not say he trusted us, he did say he was grateful for his son. I am certain that had we not taken a caritas approach, the outcome of this situation would have been much different. I would not have been able to help this father reimagine his son's life or lead him toward hope.

During this experience, I wrote down some reflections on it:

> "I could write a book of all the times that I have been mistreated. Of all the mistrust I have for this system, this hospital, this situation. You don't care for me. You don't care for my son."

> I know you don't trust me, us, them. I know you are suffering. I know you are grieving the loss of your perfect image of a son. I know you are in survival mode. I don't take it personally. I hold you in your suffering. I feel your anger without letting it in my heart.

> "I could write a book of all the ways I feel discriminated against for my skin, my knowledge, my culture."

> I hold you. I hold hope that you will find trust. Not for my needs but yours. That you will find ways to live in hope, not fear. I hold hope that we can let go of the past and see the possibilities and joy in tomorrow. I hope for you and I will not stop hoping for you until you no longer need me to do it for you but with you.

Caritas consciousness raises and holds nurses in the highest level of consciousness: love. In that space, we can hold our patients up in hope.

BROADENING THE USE OF CARITAS BEYOND THE WORKPLACE

I see a great need to spread caritas beyond our professional roles and into our homes. Caritas consciousness is not just a tool for being a better nurse; it is a tool for being a better person. I believe we are all called to show compassion to each other. Seeing the humanity in our neighbors and connecting with those around us allows caritas consciousness to expand. Viewing the world through the lens of caritas consciousness enables us to see the value in simple acts of kindness, find compassion for our own struggles and the struggles of those around us, and sense the connectedness of everything.

What we give, we receive. I give love because I need love. I offer compassion because I need compassion. Watson describes this as an expanded, deeper moral-ethical foundation. In this awakening we "open to a sense of humanity-in-relation-to-the-larger-universe, inspiring a sense of wonder, wisdom, awe and humility" (2008, p. 10). We become someone whose own self journey and discovery leads to being a light in the world—to contributing to a shared consciousness and vision of love for those in our lives and for our greater humanity and world.

FINAL REFLECTIONS

Caritas consciousness has transformed my nursing practice. It helps answer the really big questions, including why I am called to be a nurse. It ensures I always center from my heart and hold others in their wholeness and humanity until they are able to do it for themselves. It has enabled me to become literate in caring and to have the language to describe what it is that I do differently from other healthcare professionals.

Each of the 10 Caritas Processes are models for transpersonal relationships. When we practice these, we know we are in true caring relationships. These processes are also an invitation to each care provider to build a nursing practice that enables them to make a difference while still caring for themselves and flourishing in their roles. Now more than ever, we need to care for each other. We need to be the hope for others. In Watson's words, "Because we are here, we are the hope...we may be the only one who makes a difference" (Watson, 2008, p. 62).

REFERENCES

Chödrön, P. (2008). *Comfortable with uncertainty: 108 teachings on cultivating fearlessness and compassion.* Boulder, CO: Shambhala Publications.

Dass, Ram. (n.d.). Healing quotes. *Ram Dass.* Retrieved from https://www.ramdass.org/healing-quotes/

Watson, J. (2005). *Caring science as sacred science.* Philadelphia, PA: F. A. Davis Co.

Watson, J. (2008). *Nursing: The philosophy and science of caring* (rev. ed.). Boulder, CO: University Press of Colorado.

Love Is the Essence

–Nicholas J. Peterson, MSN, BSN, BA, RN,
Caritas Coach

Nick invites us to share the grace and gratitude of living as a Caritas Coach, beginning with his daily practices with his family and extending to all aspects of his work life. He shows us what it means to be human and how vulnerability, intention, engagement, and the beauty around us can be manifested in each moment–whether at a meeting, while teaching, while orienting new staff, as a student, or with a family member.

NICK'S CARITAS JOURNEY

To become a Caritas Coach is to study what it means to be a sentient being in the context of our relationships with each other and in our universe. Dr. Jean Watson's theory of Caring Science describes the relationships of humans at a vibratory level, with love at the source (2008). This is our essential nature. This is human nature. This is a loving energy.

As Caritas Coaches, we are beacons of vibratory light. Our purpose is to help nurses and other caregivers become aware of the loving energy (the light) that fuels their passion for their work and drives all that is good. This energy calms, soothes, and ultimately heals. Especially in times of stress and vulnerability, this energy naturally positions all in loving relationship with one another. We intentionally manifest loving energy, creating opportunities for transpersonal connections between ourselves and others.

Caritas Coaches are consciously aware of their vibratory power—their loving energy. They manifest opportunities to deeply connect with nurses and other colleagues. As Caritas Coaches, we are open to others. We are open to the experiences of others, listening so we can understand another's perspective. We invite the other to connect, whether by touch, spoken word, or shared space.

BEING GROUNDED IN LOVE

The Caritas Coach awakens each day to endless potential. Manifesting an open system of love and human connection often results in unpredictable and miraculous events. Watson reminds us to live in gratitude. We appreciate all the miracles of the day, starting with our breath in and out. We are not limited in our potential for gratitude. With mindfulness, we become acutely aware of a rainbow of miracles—a beautiful display of beauty, grace, and joy in our world.

To the reader, this must sound very esoteric. But in reality this way of being is quite simple. Even as I sit at my kitchen table, typing away on my laptop, I am aware of my breathing and of the quiet of the morning. I am enjoying a delicious cup of coffee and a slice of toast with peanut butter and jam. Such luxury! I can hear the sounds of my family navigating these early moments of the day—my son's feet against the floor above my head, my daughter calling out from her room to ask about the weather, my spouse putting away dishes from last night's dinner. I am filled with a sense of gratitude and peace as my day begins. It is a miracle of sorts. My heart is filled.

As I prepare for my workday I consider the meetings and administrative tasks associated with my role as a nurse educator. I think about how I want to affect my world. How will my energy manifest the environment for my day—and how I will be in that environment? I visualize coworkers and new staff. I visualize myself engaged, smiling, listening, and connecting. These thoughts and visualizations—these intentions—provide me with a sense of hope and direction. I know that when I am in an environment grounded in love, transpersonal caring relationships will manifest. I know that in the caring moment associated with transpersonal relationships, we feel loved, cared for, and connected.

Caritas affects all aspects of my work environment. During a recent clinical practice policy committee meeting to hammer out (very dry) descriptions of procedures, committee members took the opportunity to check in with each other to see how everyone was doing with their caritas practice. The committee chair, a Caritas Coach, quickly manifested a caring environment by shifting her energy to reflect a loving intention. Soon the nurses sitting around the table were chiming in about their understanding of caritas and their work. I was especially touched by one nurse who shed tears as she related a story about an emotional connection she made with one of her staff nurses. In that moment, she was supported and loved by her colleagues. Her tears were a gift—a miracle, really—that reminded me of how vulnerable we humans are. This was a caring moment—a transpersonal experience—in the midst of one of the most mundane, dry, and unemotional of nursing tasks.

IT'S ALL ABOUT HEALING

Watson believes the role of nurses has become so technical and factory-like that our purpose—our relationship to patient care—is no longer clear (2008). Yes, nurses need to understand the science, technology, diagnostics, and treatments associated with disease states to treat our patients. But to heal, nurses have an additional responsibility—one that relates to the very human elements of the patient and to one another. Watson reminds us to consider our patients, ourselves, and others in terms of "mind-body-spirit" (2008, p. 65). She observes that patients are languishing, nurses feel lost and burned out, and humanity suffers because we have lost our human connection with one another. She reminds us that the purpose of nursing is not to cure, but to heal—through human, heartfelt connections and loving-kindness.

Caring Science and its emphasis on healing inform the content of my educational endeavors as well as my way of being with my students. As a nurse educator, my focus is rarely described as healing. The objectives and outcomes for my curriculum are far more analytical and scientific. But in fact, I believe my work is all about healing. I strive to convey the Caring Science concept that the patient is more than a diseased body and the nurse is more than a technician. Both patients and nurses are composed of mind-body-spirit, and all three must be tended to.

I simply will not succeed as an educator if I don't consider the mind-body-spirit of my students. I am always aware of each student as a whole person. This becomes obvious in new employee orientation, where anxiety can run so high it commonly produces errors and tears. For me, these errors and tears are simply part of what it means to be human so I address them in a loving and caring manner. This enables new employees to lift themselves up and take in the learning experience.

As part of new employee orientation, we discuss Caring Science. This module includes a video about empathy. The purpose of this video is to move employees from an emotionally unengaged place (lecture learning) to one of heartfelt feeling and empathy, and perhaps create a sensory emotional experience. While viewing the video, students are frequently moved to tears. As the leader of this learning experience, I can allow myself to experience the video and let my tears flow. Alternatively I can remove myself from the experience so I won't have to endure the vulnerability I associate with crying or the mixed reactions I often get from my audience when they see me in this state. I always choose to endure my vulnerability. I want these newly hired nurses to see me this way so they will know it is OK to be human. It is OK to have emotions, even as professional nurses—or, as Caring Science would suggest, *because* we are professional nurses.

Transpersonal Caring Moments as Teachable Moments

Imagine a staff nurse working in one of the many ambulatory sites associated with a hospital. Lately, patients and coworkers have complained about this staff nurse to the practice manager. As the ambulatory nurse educator, I have been assigned the task of meeting with this staff nurse, observing his telephone triage in real time, and reporting my findings back to the director of nursing to consider next steps. Most likely, the dynamic between the staff nurse (who is being observed and assessed) and me (the nurse educator or authority performing the observation and assessment) will feel awkward and unbalanced and foster a real sense of vulnerability for both of us.

Before I meet with the staff nurse, I ponder my intention from the caritas perspective. I consider my feelings, my energy, and the dynamic I will bring to this exchange. I intentionally and purposefully center myself, take a moment to breathe, and quite literally think about being a loving, caring, healing energy.

I enter the space with the staff nurse with a warm smile and a kind word. I touch his shoulder or shake his hand as a gesture of support. I position myself in a nonthreatening way in the space. I inquire. I listen. I want to try to understand the wholeness of the staff nurse. I don't just want to collect data on his phone triage skills; I also need to understand the entirety of the staff nurse—his feelings and what is happening in a broader sense.

Often in these moments of inquiry a transpersonal caring moment occurs (Watson, 2008). It is in these moments when I open myself at a vibratory level and am able to listen deeply, understand, and explore that I can meet the other where they are in body, mind, and spirit. Often in these moments, one person is sharing something very personal that may make him or her feel vulnerable, and the other person is participating in that moment, mindful only of the first person's need to share it. These are the transpersonal caring experiences in my role as nurse educator.

Loving-Kindness and Connection

Watson invites us on a journey to heal. The caring theory describes the healing power of loving-kindness. The first of the 10 Caritas Processes speaks of loving-kindness for self and others (Watson, 2008). In this first process, Watson provides permission to intentionally connect with loving-kindness toward ourselves as individuals. Through meditation and other self-care initiatives we discover the self that may need to be nurtured deep inside. If we pay close attention in this process, some of us discover a light that may have been subdued that can shine only through self-reflection, surrender, forgiveness, mindfulness, and loving-kindness. In this light, many of us discover talents, passions, and confidence that propel us forward. For me, this process is exciting and sometimes anxiety provoking—a time filled with hope and opportunity.

Of course, there is a direct correlation between one's experience of self—the loving and healing energy in one's personal life—and one's professional experience, evolution, and development. We can view the world only via the lens through which we are looking at any given time. For a nurse who encounters the gamut of extreme human experiences every day, who bears witness to and participates in great tragedies and miraculously joyful moments, the aim must be to orient the self toward balance and to an openness to the human experience with the capacity to love and care for others. Moving toward equilibrium in life—in all aspects of life—provides a safe and strong foundation for the nurse to work.

If we all agree that nurses are more than technicians, that their role is to promote healing, then nurses must—to the degree they can—be as healthy and resilient as possible. "Health" is subjective and uniquely one's own, but the impact of loving-kindness on health is proven. Whether for themselves or their patients, each nurse's ability to manifest the life-giving, biogenic force of loving-kindness is integral to his or her healing effectiveness. When we feel "healthy," our lens is clear and the world is full of possibilities.

This has led me to a place of joy at work. I can intentionally manifest the energy of loving-kindness and accessibility. My connections with colleagues and staff nurses have a deeper potential to reflect caring and love. It has been powerful. Indeed, in this environment, I have even been able to complete my master's degree in nursing education and am pursuing certification in the area of nursing professional development.

Considering Our Own Narrative

Self-reflection leads to self-awareness. It provides an opportunity for us to consider our own narrative. Critically considering our actions—how we respond in a given situation—provides the opportunity to learn and grow from our own experiences and actions.

I use self-reflection in daily journaling. I believe this process reveals a trajectory for my life. Writing down my feelings, observations, hopes, and dreams has led me to make significant changes in my personal life, such as the following:

- I am a talented painter but I hadn't painted in 5 years—since my spouse and I adopted children (my excuse). Reflecting on this, I realized I missed painting. I then realized I *can* paint and I created a path to paint again.

- I am studying the power of love, kindness, and caring, and I want to manifest this in my personal life as well as in my professional one. I engage in meditative experiences and spiritual pursuits. I reengage in my spiritual community by attending church on a regular basis. I connect with other people who are interested in understanding the mysteries of the universe, their connection to the universal consciousness, and the interconnectedness of all things.

- To access loving-kindness for others, I must love and take care of myself. This starts with my physical self. I think about my diet—about healthy foods, about enjoying my food, and about making food choices that support my personal equilibrium. In addition, I have increased the amount of physical exercise I engage in. This is not easy because of back problems but I get stronger every day. As I get older this provides me with hope and confidence.

- It used to be that my work life overwhelmed all other aspects of my life. Although it was often very rewarding, this caused me to feel separated from opportunities for personal reflection and growth. In becoming a Caritas Coach, my relationship with work has evolved. I have made more time to be in relationship with my family, my friends, and my greater community.

FINAL REFLECTIONS

We invite others to sit at this table. This table is a banquet with many familiar and comforting foods as well as new things to try. At this banquet, the food nourishes the body, mind, and spirit. Not only is the individual nourished, but with our awareness of the interconnectedness of all living things—and our connection to the universal consciousness—the whole world is made healthier. The cost to sit at this table is no more than our ability to live with an intention of loving-kindness and to pursue the spiritual resources that we all can access within ourselves.

REFERENCE

Watson, J. (2008). *Nursing: The philosophy and science of caring* (rev. ed.). Boulder, CO: University Press of Colorado.

4

CARITAS PRAXIS

Nursing as a Sacred Act of Caring: Practicing with an Open Mind and Open Heart

–Katherine E. Belategui, BSN, RN, Caritas Coach

In this chapter, Katherine explores how Caring Science has transformed the way she thinks, practices, and interacts in her environment. She explains how her thinking has shifted from focusing on tasks to focusing on her heart. This places love at the foundation of her practice and positively radiates into her environment. Katherine also shares *presencing* exercises and other reflective practices that keep her rooted in love. Finally, Katherine provides clinical examples of how this carries over to the care of patients and interactions with colleagues.

KATHERINE'S CARITAS JOURNEY

"Feelings come and go like clouds in a windy sky. Conscious breathing is my anchor."

–Thich Nhat Hanh

Becoming a Caritas Coach was a beautiful, transformational journey. It taught me to see how caring and love exist in every context if we are willing to shine a light and see them. To me, being a Caritas Coach means being the light that others draw from during life's most grueling moments. To become a Caritas Coach, one must learn to practice forgiveness, compassion, surrender, and gratitude (Watson, 2008). To do the work of a Caritas Coach, one must practice with an open heart and a clear mind.

In 2016 I attended the International Caritas Consortium (ICC). At this annual 2-day interactive and collaborative professional practice gathering, individuals actively engage in applying Caring Science. Afterward, I felt renewed and inspired by all the nurses I met from all over the world who embody caritas and who infuse Caring Science into their practice. Perhaps more importantly, I was relieved to learn that other nurses also face a dilemma that I find particularly challenging: "Nurses are torn between the human caring model of nursing that attracted them to the profession and the task oriented biomedical model and institutional demands that consumes their practice time" (Watson & Foster, 2003, p. 360). Seeing caritas nurses recognize and address this challenge at the ICC prompted me to reflect on how Caring Science has transformed my thinking, my practice, and the way I interact with my environment. I am so proud to be a nurse—to be part of a sacred profession that has the power to create and bear witness to life's greatest miracles!

Thinking and Practicing Caritas

Before studying Caring Science, my thinking and practice involved a nurse-patient relationship based on setting and attaining goals. "Health" and "healing" were assessed by the success of the nurse-patient dyad in achieving goals. This mindset allowed me to slip into a robotic way of thinking, interacting, and being—skating over the living and breathing human patient.

Discovering Caring Science and becoming a caritas nurse shifted my thinking from a task-oriented focus to a heart focus. Practicing from my heart puts love—the greatest power of all—at the forefront of my practice. Being heart-centered grounds me and enables me to practice with intention, mindfulness, and equanimity. Shifting to a heart-centered practice has also changed the way I view the nurse-patient relationship. I now celebrate this relationship as a fluid, giving and receiving relationship. I do not judge this relationship or quantify it with outcomes. I pay special attention to it and celebrate the miracles that occur as a result of creating human-to-human connections.

I see the nurse-patient relationship as existing between two energy beings that perceive, interact, and grow. When one views humans as energy beings, it becomes clear how nurses *are* the environment. We hold the opportunity to change the environment around us by practicing mindfulness and acting from a heart-centered place.

I work as a nurse in charge of a small 10-room unit—a circular pod with an open-concept nurses' station in the middle. It is not uncommon for four or five different interdisciplinary teams to visit the unit during the day. At the same time, nurses weave in and out of patient rooms, attend the interdisciplinary huddle, and patients and family members often walk around the pod. In this environment, it is easy to quickly transmit energy from one person to the next. When that energy is negative, it is palpable.

I have learned to make small changes to this environment by changing my energy. I used to walk quickly—as fast as I could—to save time. Now I slow down. I walk at a slower-than-normal pace to shift the energy toward calmness. I also speak softly to minimize noise in the unit. Finally, I used to review my patient's report sheet and then knock on the patient's door as I entered his or her room. Although this practice did result in a brief pause, it put my agenda at the center of my attention. As a Caritas Coach, I have learned that clearing my mind opens my heart, places the needs of the person in my care at the forefront, enables me to be authentically present, and allows caring moments to occur. Now I center myself before entering the patient's space. I pause at the patient's door, apply hand sanitizer, take a deep breath, knock on the door, pause again, and then enter the room.

Whenever I find myself being swept away by the business of the unit, I focus my attention back to my body and my heart to remain present and mindful of each person in my care and his or her needs.

Exploring the Patient's Frame of Reference

I care for neuroscience patients on an intermediate medical-surgical unit. Nearly all my patients suffer from some sort of organic or in-organic cognitive deficit. Because of this, they often have an altered perception of reality. As their nurse, I must be able to enter their reality and explore their world from their frame of reference in order for transpersonal caring moments to occur.

I cared for an elderly woman I'll call Mrs. B, who had a history of dementia. She was admitted after suffering a stroke that had left her with hemiparesis, vision loss, and worsening confusion. Given her prognosis, her family transitioned her to end-of-life care. Her care plan included only measures to make her comfortable. She was not a typical end-of-life patient, however. She could still eat and drink and move from the bed to the chair.

Mrs. B. was from Canada and spoke only French. I called in an interpreter. But due to her stroke, Mrs. B.'s speech had become too garbled for the interpreter to understand. This presented a problem. How would I know what Mrs. B. wanted to eat and when? How would I know if she was more comfortable in the bed or the chair? Most importantly, how would I know when she was in pain? I started observing Mrs. B. closely. My intention was to wait for an invitation from her to intervene. It was as if the two of us were dancing. She was the leader and I followed. I used her body language and her reactions to my interventions to learn exactly what she wanted.

We never spoke a word. We couldn't. We didn't understand each other in that way. But I was surprised by how much I got to know her through our dance. I learned that when she was hungry, she tried to get out of bed. I learned that she liked to sleep in the chair in the afternoon and to be lifted back into bed at midnight. I learned that she loved bananas on her pancakes. I learned that when she was in pain she clenched her left fist. Through authentic presence, I was able to create a human-to-human connection with Mrs. B. and build a transpersonal caring relationship despite her cognitive, communication, and sensory deficits.

This fall my hospital hosted a patient education committee meeting to explore the topic of frame of reference. The committee was composed of inpatient and outpatient nurses, nurse educators, nursing directors, and nurse executives dedicated to enhancing and strengthening patient education modalities. I was asked to lead a discussion during the meeting on Caring Science concepts and on Caritas Process 7: "Engaging in genuine teaching-learning experiences within context of caring relationship—attend to whole person and subjective meaning; attempt to stay within other's frame of reference (evolve toward 'coaching' role vs. conventional imparting of information)" (Watson, 2008, p. 125). During the discussion, I asked the group to share stories about how they stayed within their patients' frame of reference—specifically patients who leave the hospital against medical advice. The goal was to come up with a collective strategy to help patients who have had negative experiences that have prevented them from being open to love, peace, caring, and healing. One nurse asked me, "As a

Caritas Coach, how do you deal with these situations?" I used this question as an opportunity to explain how Caring Science and caring literacy have changed my way of being and ways of interacting with others, my environment, and my nursing practice. As much as it pains me to see a patient leave against medical advice, I know that as a nurse I have a unique opportunity to create a transpersonal connection with that patient and to help him or her feel loved and known. Therefore, in these situations, my goal shifts to sustaining an altruistic-human connection so that this patient knows he or she is always welcome back to the hospital and that we will always meet the patient with open arms when he or she is in need.

FOSTERING TRANSPERSONAL CARING RELATIONSHIPS

Sometimes it is difficult to sustain transpersonal caring and practice from a heart-centered place when faced with challenging and stressful situations. Journaling and self-reflection have led me to use mantras as a way of grounding myself. I put this approach to the test while caring for a young patient who had undergone back surgery to relieve chronic lower-back pain. After his surgery, the patient's pain became worse. Our care team was having trouble devising a plan that relieved his pain without sedating him.

One morning the boy's mother visited the hospital and asked to speak with me because I was the nurse in charge of her son's care. As I walked to the nurses' station to meet her, I saw her from afar— tense, pacing, scanning the unit. Her negative energy was palpable. I took a deep breath, relaxed my posture, slowly approached her, and introduced myself. "Ha! You have got to be kidding me!" she cried. "You can't possibly be old enough to know what you're doing. No wonder my son is in so much pain!" The unit went still. The silence sent goose bumps down my neck. My heart raced. Her words burned through me. I realized that in this moment, I had to two choices. I could take her actions personally and become defensive.

Or I could adopt a nonjudgmental attitude from a heart-centered place.

I decided to do the latter. I took a breath—deeper than normal—which healed the wound in my heart. I held onto that breath and space and thought about love. Then I exhaled. As I did, I recalled one of my mantras: "I am on her team. I am here to help her. I am on her side." Calling on this mantra enabled me to respond from a heart-centered place. It reminded me that it was a privilege to be her son's nurse. It reminded me that in that moment I was the only person who could relieve her suffering. My breath empowered me to see this woman simply as a mother who was looking out for her son and acting from a place of love.

I responded to the woman by first acknowledging her pain and her son's suffering. I assured her that I was suffering with them and that I was on their team in this battle to defeat chronic pain. Then I took her hand and looked her in the eye. As I held her gaze, I continued to breathe, slightly deeper than normal, and to repeat my mantra in my mind. In that space, time froze for a moment. I could tell she was faced with the same two choices. Finally, the energy changed. The woman apologized to me. After that, we worked as a team to heal her son.

This story is about mantras, but it's also about breathing. I use HeartMath to guide and sustain me through difficult moments. Consciously changing my breathing pattern with "quick coherences" helps me become more self-aware and authentically present in each moment. I use HeartMath during difficult conversations—for example, talking with relatives about care for their critically ill family member. I breathe as a way of grounding myself and releasing my personal beliefs about a situation so I can be authentically present without being emotionally withdrawn.

CARING LITERACY AND THE "L WORD"

Nurses refer to their "intuition" as a source of strength and "way of knowing" when caring for patients (Young, 1987). This phenomenon stems from experience and connections created with patients. Young (1987) defines nursing intuition as "a process whereby the nurse knows something about a patient that cannot be verbalized, that is verbalized with difficulty, or for which the source cannot be determined" (Young, 1987). Others refer to nursing intuition as a "sixth sense" (Zander, 2007, p. 9).

Traditionally, intuitive knowledge has not been considered valuable because it cannot be logically explained. Studying Caring Science and becoming a Caritas Coach have shown me how caring literacy can be used to describe nursing intuition and to explain how it can help to reestablish nursing as a caring-healing profession. Watson (2008) notes the importance of caring literacies and ontologies in creating balance in a technology-driven, bio-focused practice (p. 24). Identifying, describing, and naming ontological caring-healing practices through caring literacy enables us to research, document, and replicate these practices—and nursing intuition along with them (p. 25).

As a new Caritas Coach, I recognized the importance of naming caritas phenomena to illuminate their existence and to celebrate that existence within the individual and the environment. To introduce Caring Science and caring literacy to the nursing practice on my unit, I created 10 posters—one for each Caritas Process—to hang above the entrance to each patient room. I intentionally hung the posters before introducing any Caring Science concepts to my colleagues. The next morning I studied my staff's reactions as they rounded the corner onto the unit. Some nurses read the processes aloud. Others expressed how they connected with a certain process. And everyone appreciated the eloquent language. One nurse asked, "What is this about—a nursing theory?" Another nurse replied, "This is what we do. This is nursing."

I was not surprised to find that some nurses were shocked by the use of the "L word"—love—in the Caritas Processes. That word is rarely used in healthcare. However, it was not long before I began to witness small miracles in day-to-day interactions with my colleagues. Suddenly, nurses began to talk about using authentic presence and practicing with intention as a way of creating a healing environment for their patients—something they had always done but never expressed. Was it possible that the explicit use of the word gave my colleagues permission to rediscover, reignite, and again embody the reason they became nurses?

Ask nurses why they chose the profession—why they chose to dedicate their life to serving others—and they will eagerly tell you. Every nurse has a story that lives inside his or her heart. Each nurse's story is a unique testimony to the desire to provide relief for and heal those who suffer. Take mine. I became a nurse to heal, to help others celebrate the miracles that life brings, and to cultivate and sustain human-to-human connections. Nurses summon these stories during challenging shifts and difficult moments to reignite their inner light and source of being. Sadly, however, it is becoming more and more difficult to access these stories—this inner light—in our linear, technology-saturated work environment, where outcomes and health are tracked by data rather than altruistic and compassionate human experiences. As Watson moves nursing back to a caring-healing model, her Caritas Processes guide and sustain me.

One of the greatest gifts I have received as a nurse came from a patient I cared for named Ardita. Ardita had given up her career as a pediatric neuroscience nurse in Albania to move to the United States to care for her daughter who had been diagnosed with cancer. After suffering a small stroke, Ardita was placed in my care. The first day I took care of Ardita, her husband, daughters, and grandchildren stayed at her bedside. "I want to go home," she said to them over and over. "Please do anything you can to get me home as soon as possible." But Ardita couldn't leave until her neurovascular surgeon informed us as to whether she needed a carotid endarterectomy or not.

Ardita was a nurse—a caregiver at heart. I could see she was having trouble surrendering to the situation. I told Ardita that I understood she was anxious to return home to care for her family and that being in the hospital made her sad. "Katie," she replied. "You are always smiling. For me, that is enough. I will be alright."

The next morning, when I stepped onto the unit, I saw Ardita waving at me from her bed. I went straight to her room. She told me she was going in for surgery that day. She seemed worried. She frowned and asked me, "Will I make it?" In this moment, I could see she was vulnerable. "Together we can have hope that everything will be OK," I said. "If you get nervous when you are in the pre-op area, think of me, and know that you are in my heart and I am sending you positive thoughts."

A short time later, surgical technicians arrived to take Ardita to surgery. I held her hand and wished her luck. She smiled at me. "Katie, I love you!" she said. I was filled with joy. Did a patient really just tell me she loved me? Before I could respond, Ardita pronounced, "Yes! I said I love you!"

EMBRACING ALL WAYS OF KNOWING

Some time ago, before I became a Caritas Coach, I took care of a patient who was an artist. He painted the most beautiful New England landscapes. As he showed me photos of his work on his phone, I said to him, "You are far more creative than I am!" "Oh no," he replied. "Nurses are the most creative beings of all! Nurses find ways to solve any problem, big or small. They have to be creative!"

As I look back on this moment, I am reminded of Caritas Process 6: "Creative use of self and all ways of knowing/being/doing as part of the caring process (engaging in artistry of caring-healing practices)" (Watson, 2008, p. 107). As a caritas nurse, I recognize the importance of creatively blending scientific information and human values. I like to think of this blend as "nursing knowledge"—that special information and insight that nurses bring to the table. We get this information from "all ways of knowing," including collecting empirical data, such as vital signs; conducting physical assessments; and learning about our patients and their values by practicing authentic presence and listening with intention. This synthesis of information is a creative process because it draws upon "all ways of knowing" and thinking about the patient as a whole.

Watson (2008) recognizes that "knowledge alone does not mean understanding" and that "even understanding...does not necessarily include insight, reflection, and wisdom" (p. 109). The caritas nurse, as the artist pointed out, is a creative problem-solver. The caritas nurse reflects upon "all ways of knowing" and on his or her highest level of consciousness to heal patients.

Final Reflections

Perhaps the most transformational gift that my caritas journey has given me so far is the discovery that love truly is the greatest power of all. Caring Science has shown me how to open my heart, to practice with unconditional loving-kindness for every patient, and to turn some of life's worst moments into miracles. Caring for patients during their most vulnerable moments is an honor and a privilege. I am so proud to be a nurse and to have the opportunity to practice nursing as a sacred act of caring.

References

Watson, J. (2008). *Nursing: The philosophy and science of caring* (rev. ed.). Boulder, CO: University Press of Colorado.

Watson, J., & Foster, R. (2003). The attending nurse caring model: Integrating theory, evidence and advanced caring-healing therapeutics for transforming professional practice. *Journal of Clinical Nursing, 12*(3), 360–365. doi:10.1046/j.1365-2702.2003.00774.x

Young, C. (1987). Intuition and nursing process. *Holistic Nursing Practice 1*(3), 52–62.

Zander, P. E. (2007). Ways of knowing in nursing: The historical evolution of a concept. *Journal of Theory Construction & Testing, 11*(1), 7–11.

CARITAS COACH LITERACY: SUSTAINING LOVING-KINDNESS FOR SELF AND OTHERS

-JOSEPH GIOVANNONI, DNP, APRN, CARITAS COACH, WCSI POST-DOCTORAL SCHOLAR

I n this chapter, Joseph discusses how his ability to remain connected to the universal field of love through heart-centered practices and equanimity enables him to create a healing environment for those he cares for. He shares his own journey of self-discovery and self-love—a journey that has enabled him to tap into his inner wisdom and the courage to face his own humanity—and how it has affected his transpersonal relationships and self-care in his practice.

JOSEPH'S CARITAS JOURNEY

I was born in Italy shortly after World War II and lived there until I was 13 years old. I was familiar with the Latin word *caritas* and its religious connotations of charity and mercy. My family was very poor. My parents often had to rely on the charity of others.

When I was introduced to Dr. Jean Watson's Caring Science theory, her elucidation of caritas expanded my consciousness to a higher level of knowing about the nature of our humanity and our sense of self. It provided a guiding light to a higher level of being as a professional nurse. Watson uses caritas to represent "charity and compassion, generosity of spirit. It connotes something very fine, indeed, something precious that needs to be cultivated and sustained" (Watson, 2008, p. 39).

BEING A CARITAS COACH

Caritas nurses view nursing as a sacred covenant to alleviate the suffering of humanity. They understand that "love is the highest level of consciousness and the greatest source of all healing in the world" (Watson, 2008, p. 40). Love is universal energy that interconnects all of humanity. The Caritas Coach embodies this mindset. The expanded consciousness of the Caritas Coach enables them to view all of creation as sacred and interconnected. All human beings belong to an infinite source that unites us (Watson, 2008; Levinas, 1969). Compassion, human caring, love, and empathy emerge when we are mindful of our oneness with everything. This opens our heart to be present and nonjudgmental, ready to extend loving-kindness to the self and other.

Those of us in the nursing profession must avoid using love, compassion, and human caring as buzzwords—often seen in health agency advertisements or mission statements—to promote a personal agenda. The health-science professional must embody caring and compassion in the delivery of care. A Caritas Coach personifies heart-centered consciousness, caritas consciousness, and an awareness that who he or she is extends beyond being an individual, a person, or a divided self with a personal agenda. The Caritas Coach contemplates what it means to reside in a unitary field of consciousness (Watson, 2008; Levinas, 1969). It means to be present, to discern, to cherish, to appreciate, and to give special loving attention to everything presented to them. Caritas reminds us to cultivate, sustain, and embody compassion for self and others by maintaining generosity of spirit—by knowing that every encounter is an opportunity to sustain our own and others' humanity with loving-kindness.

A Caritas Coach is mindful that a patient is not a sick, broken body that needs fixing. We must sustain and support each patient's humanity. This means understanding that beyond the body is the extension of the universal mind of love. This begins with sustaining our own humanity by identifying with the unitary field of consciousness. It is a conscious repeated understanding that the greatest source of healing is love. This is a repeated practice of being present in the moment, nonjudgmental, and compassionate when listening to another's story.

I am a forensic nurse in private practice. For the past 35 years, I have treated adjudicated sex abusers and victims of sexual assault. To be effective in my forensic work, I must be willing to enter the darkness of my own humanity to help others surface from their darkness into the light. As a child, I was sexually assaulted by an adult stranger. My competence as a forensic nurse was proportional to my courage and ability to explore, acknowledge, and address my own wounding (Giovannoni, 2016). This meant revisiting the validity of long-held beliefs and prejudices that separated me from others, recognizing and restructuring negative judgments toward myself and others with compassion and forgiveness, and simply letting go of learned fearful core beliefs that I often projected onto others. It meant realizing that thoughts and beliefs that have informed our personality are often founded in fear. These separate us from others.

As a Caritas Coach, I nurture a vision of union and I focus on my interconnectedness with everything. I am mindful to forgive my judgments that separate me from another. This process of addressing negative feelings, fear, and anger can be challenging. When I recognize negativity in myself, I engage in self-acceptance. Then I let go with self-forgiveness. I remind myself to forgive my misperceptions of others and to remain open to a deeper understanding of both myself and the other. When I witness suffering or injustice and my anger surfaces, I reset equanimity by breathing in and saying, "I know that anger is within me," and then breathing out and saying, "I am peaceful with my anger and I release it."

When I accept that I am interconnected with everything, those who cross my path often mirror what I need to do to heal and forgive within myself. What needs to be forgiven is often mirrored but disguised in another's behavior. Their behavior often calls up deep emotions that relate to my own fears and anger, which are attached to past experiences.

CREATING A HEALING ENVIRONMENT

I mentioned that I am a forensic nurse. Many of my patients have co-morbidities such as drug addiction, domestic violence, or mental health disorders. Needless to say, this work can be very stressful. It's easy to burn out. Interacting with disgruntled patients who do not take responsibility for their actions and who blame others (including their victims) for their legal predicaments can trigger frustration and anxiety. It is easy to close my heart—to view these patients as less than human. But doing so dehumanizes them...and me.

Since I became a Caritas Coach, the light of caritas consciousness has entered through a crack in my self-protective shell. Caritas has helped me open my compassionate heart. Caring Science informs me of the powerful caring-healing practices of heart-centered breathing, reminding me that my heart is much more than a pump (Rosch, 2015).

I try to consciously start all my interviews with caritas consciousness. It helps me be present in the moment and to observe and discern without judgment. It facilitates radiant energetic compassion. It sets a calming, safe, and healing environment for my patients, helping them to be more open and cooperative. Remaining mindful of Caritas Process 1, "Practicing loving-kindness and equanimity for self and other" (Watson, 2008, p. 47), is essential in this work. Loving-kindness starts with the breath—with consciously breathing into the heart, which has neural connections that communicate directly with the amygdala, the emotional center in the brain. Anger is triggered in the amygdala. This can result in a cascade of neurohormones such as cortisone that are detrimental to our organs. I find deep breathing—extending heart-centered loving-kindness with self-affirmations on the in breath, such as "May I be safe, may I be healed, may I be helpful," and the out breath, such as "Let go of fear and forgive"—to be extremely helpful in combating this.

Offering care and compassion to aggressive individuals who have *not* behaved in a caring manner toward others might seem counterintuitive. But I believe it is a privilege to be available to, to be present for, and to extend loving-kindness to those who have behaved unlovingly. This does not mean I don't hold my patients responsible and accountable for their actions or that I don't attempt to correct their core beliefs that separate them from others. But if I want to facilitate healing and learning, then I must provide a loving and compassionate environment. If I want them to change, then I must embody compassion and human caring. By extending loving-kindness and forgiveness, we can help others see the errors in their thinking and correct the core beliefs that caused their behavior. Responding to them with anger or indifference would only emulate the inhumanity of their behavior. Being mindful that we all belong to the infinite field of universal love—holding their humanity sacred— keeps my judgments at bay.

As I continue to integrate human caring and compassion into my forensic practice, my relationships with my patients and colleagues have improved. I measure the efficacy of human caring and compassion in my practice by the authentic power I experience with each transpersonal caring moment. For example, being present and heart-centered with an angry or frustrated patient and allowing him or her to express negative emotions verbally (Caritas Process 5) can turn a negative interaction into a positive and collaborative relationship. Often, the patient's facial expression will soften and his or her body becomes relaxed and at ease. Seeing beyond the shadow of the self-centered individual and responding with loving-kindness facilitates Caritas Process 4, "Developing and sustaining a helping-trusting, authentic caring relationship" (Watson, 2008, p. 71).

HOLDING SACRED SPACE TO MAINTAIN LOVING-KINDNESS FOR SELF AND OTHERS

For many, feeling helpless or afraid fuels their need for power and triggers violence. When we ignore or disavow that we are interconnected and part of a unified mind, our humanity falls prey to the ego's divided self. When our needs are not met, we tend to engage in negative thinking that justifies our desire for immediate gratification and become vulnerable to addictive patterns of behavior. I had to be willing to go into the dark corridors of my own ego, practice self-forgiveness, and be present without judgment to help guide my patients to the light of their own humanity. To be a role model of human caring we must carry the torch of compassion for the self first, to help others return to the light of love.

My wife, Jill, is the administrator of my practice. She has participated in all aspects of my Caritas Coach training. In our clinic, she often collectively experiences the interactions I have with difficult patients. She is very poetic and shared with me a reflection of her own experience when I was interviewing a challenging and angry patient during an evaluation for the courts. This individual repeatedly blamed everyone else for his own bad choices, which had caused harm to others and consequently to himself, being a registered sex offender. It was important for me to recognize my fears, negative thoughts, judgments, and the anger that I felt rising up within my body. I gently challenged my own negative thoughts and emerged with compassion, forgiveness, gratitude, and reverence. I focused on breathing into my heart as I listened to his negative emotionality and on not allowing myself to descend into the abyss of anger and helplessness. I was not aware that Jill was also experiencing the biocidic energy field that permeated through the wall into her office in the next room. She poetically illuminated her own experience of this incident.

DARK CLOUD OF DEPRESSION
By Jill Giovannoni

He arrived for his session

He's none too happy about being here

The energy I described is like wrapping yourself with a blanket in a hot desert

I feel prickly all over

Feeling as if I rolled in cactus

The air is thick and moves slowly

I feel the darkness wants to take over

The calm before the storm

The sun fades fighting to break through the clouds

The cloud tries to block the light of happiness and love

I struggle to feel even one little teeny tiny sun ray

My energetic field feels heavy pulling me down

I try to keep afloat

It pulls me down and tries to keep me in the negative energy flow

I breathe and say that I choose not to allow

the negativity to envelop me

Clear my space and fill it with love
Breathing in love and peace
Breathing out what weighs me down
I am floating freely through the light and clouds of love, peace, and joy

EMBRACING ALL FORMS OF KNOWING

Since completing my Caritas Coach education in 2014, I have continued to develop caritas literacy. I have embraced all forms of knowing and creative scholarship to further expand the phenomena of human caring, healing, and being human. The value of philosophical concepts such as love, non-physical phenomena, intentionality, and forgiveness cannot be dismissed from forensic nursing.

One way I learn is by teaching. I have developed and delivered workshops to probation officers and forensic nurses to help them lower stress with mindful practices. I have taught nationally and internationally and at various conferences. The ethics of belonging to an infinite field of universal love is the starting point for Caring Science (Watson, 2008). I teach this principle in my workshops.

I have also taken on the challenge to gain a deeper understanding of the causes of violence and develop creative solutions (Caritas Process 6) by collaborating with colleagues. Being aware of and relinquishing any personal agenda facilitates cooperation toward collective wisdom. To effectively address violence, we must consider the following Caring Science principles:

- All creation is sacred and connected.

- All humans belong to the infinite source that unites us.

- Every person has the right to receive compassionate care.

- All humans are entitled to be free of tyranny, violation, and abuse.

BECOMING A COMPASSIONATE CARING HEALER

As healthcare professionals, we are constantly confronted with pain and suffering. Caring for others makes us vulnerable to compassion fatigue and vicarious trauma (Elias & Haj-Yahia, 2016; Ennis & Home, 2003; Hatcher & Noakes, 2010). Signs of compassion fatigue include anger, cynicism, and indifference, and signs of vicarious trauma are hypervigilance, helplessness, detachment, difficulty managing emotions and establishing boundaries, and experiencing problems with relationships (Van Dernoot Lipsky & Burk, 2009).

In my daily practice, I review victim statements. I constantly remind myself that being exposed to people who are suffering can have negative emotional, physical, and psychological effects on my well-being (Perlman & Saakvitne, 1995). It's imperative that I identify and mediate my own individual risk factors for compassion fatigue and vicarious trauma as well as for burnout (Rothschild & Rand, 2006). Self-awareness is critical. I cannot afford to overlook the daily stress I encounter and how it affects me.

I have repeatedly asked myself why I choose to do the kind of work I do. I've found that gaining a deeper understanding of my purpose and the choices I make requires loving-kindness and the courage to explore, acknowledge, and address my own personal wounding. I must be conscious of my own traumas—including sexual assault—and how those experiences have informed my choice to become a nurse, to study psychology, to become a sex therapist, and to become a sex-offender treatment specialist.

Our ability to help people change self-destructive behaviors that contribute to the suffering of others as well as themselves depends on the development of a transpersonal caring relationship. This is not always easy with individuals who do not think they have a problem or who do not want my help. I find that shifting the focus to my patients' strengths, rather than continuously focusing on their crime, helps them become more mindful of their loving nature and respectful of others' boundaries. Using mindfulness practices such as deep heart-centered breathing before cognitive behavioral group sessions has facilitated presence and authenticity among group members as well as support, connections, and caring moments.

The efficacy of our professional skills—regardless of specialty—is proportionally related to our being and becoming a conscious, caring, and compassionate healer. Caritas consciousness occurs when we are heart-centered and sustain our humanity and the humanity of others—even those who terrorize others. When informed by Caring Science, nursing is a sacred profession (Watson, 2005). It goes beyond the mechanical and technical skills of science. This requires a deep faith in the notion that we are connected with a universal source of consciousness of love that transcends time, space, and physicality—a consciousness that is omnipresent, infinite, and ultimately one with everything. To access this we must expand our five senses to a multisensory consciousness, moving beyond the divided ego self to a higher self that is interconnected with a unitary field of consciousness.

FINAL REFLECTIONS

The philosopher Joseph Campbell once said, "The privilege of a lifetime is being who you are" (Campbell, 1995). This requires self-awareness and self-reflection. These practices also facilitate my caritas consciousness. To cultivate this consciousness, I make time to be still and pause. I breathe into my heart and intentionally visualize infinite source. My eyes extend like a telescope into the infinity of the unified mind of the universe. In this mindful space it becomes easier for me to observe and discern without judgment what is being presented to me. Intuitively I become aware of any personal agenda and I practice letting go. I seek a deep sense of humility, gratitude, and compassion for myself, and I am more available to forgive. Being conscious of my breath, I open my heart to be authentically present to extend loving-kindness to others and to be open to the collective wisdom of those who seek the truth about the nature of our being.

Being very visual, I often create posters during the process of introspection, reflection, and centering to illuminate my self-awareness. These posters promote personal healing and facilitate compassion for myself and those who are entrusted into my care. In closing I will share the words of one of these posters with you:

> I was given a lamp to go on a difficult journey that involved a grueling and dangerous descent into the personal and collective shadow.
>
> It was most empowering because it brought the light of deep understanding of the evolution of the human ego.
>
> We are empowered when we empty ourselves of our false concepts and attachments.
>
> Then we can return to our divine grace.

REFERENCES

Campbell, J. (1995). *Reflections on the art of living: A Joseph Campbell companion* (D. Osbon, Ed.). New York, NY: Harper Perennial.

Elias, H., & Haj-Yahia, M. M. (2016). On the lived experience of sex offenders' therapists: Their perceptions of intrapersonal and interpersonal consequences and patterns of coping. *Journal of Interpersonal Violence*, April. doi:10.1177/0886260516646090

Ennis, L., & Home, S. (2003). Predicting psychological distress in sex offender therapists. *Sexual Abuse: A Journal of Research and Treatment, 15*(2), 149–157.

Giovannoni, J. (2016). Egoless & interconnected: Suspending judgment to embrace heart-centered healthcare. In W. Rosa (Ed.), *Nurses as leaders: Evolutionary visions of leadership* (Chapter 19). New York, NY: Springer Publishing Company.

Hatcher, R., & Noakes, S. (2010). Working with sex offenders: The impact on Australian treatment providers. *Psychology, Crime & Law, 16*(1–2), 145–167.

Levinas, E. (1969). *Totality and infinity: An essay on exteriority*. Pittsburgh, PA: Duquesne University Press.

Perlman, L. A., & Saakvitne, K. W. (1995). *Trauma and the therapist: Countertransference and vicarious traumatization in psychotherapy with incest survivors*. New York, NY: W. W. Norton & Co.

Rosch, P. (2015). The heart is much more than a pump. In M. Dahlitz & G. Hall (Eds.), *An issue of the heart: The neuropsychotherapist special issue* (pp. 1–13). Brisbane, AU: Dahlitz Media.

Rothschild, B., & Rand, M. L. (2006). *Help for the helper: The psychophysiology of compassion fatigue and vicarious trauma*. New York, NY: W. W. Norton & Co.

Van Dernoot Lipsky, L., & Burk, C. (2009). *Trauma stewardship: An everyday guide to caring for self while caring for others*. Oakland, CA: Berrett-Koehler Publishers Co.

Watson, J. (2005). *Caring science as sacred science*. Philadelphia, PA: F. A. Davis Co.

Watson, J. (2008). *Nursing: The philosophy and science of caring* (rev. ed.). Boulder, CO: University Press of Colorado.

CARITAS COACH REFLECTIONS

–HEIDI J. HAGLE, RN, HN-BC, CARITAS COACH

In this chapter, Heidi discusses how she overcame her fear of the unknown through the lessons of loving-kindness and reflection, and how she learned that taking care of herself helps her to more authentically care for others. Heidi also shares the caring-healing routines that have guided her practice and how she has implemented them to decrease stress and improve care for pre-surgical patients.

HEIDI'S CARITAS JOURNEY

When I was asked by nursing leadership at St. John Hospital to apply for the Caritas Coach Education Program (CCEP), I was filled with joy and immediately accepted. I was so grateful to have the opportunity to start on the journey to become a Caritas Coach.

At the beginning of the program I had many fears—fears of the unknown and of what would be expected of me during and after the program. But after meeting my fellow cohort I felt at ease, as they shared a similar fear of the unknown. And when I started the first session, the caritas faculty welcomed me with loving-kindness.

The 6-month program passed by very quickly. As the weeks progressed, participating in online discussion boards and sharing our reflective assignments helped my cohort to develop relationships and build our own caritas community. I learned that I needed to take care of myself and that before I could authentically care for another, I needed to fully examine my own deep unresolved feelings. My own self-care had long been pushed aside, but the continued guidance and support from my mentors encouraged me to be mindful in caring for myself. This guidance and support also enabled me to develop and complete a project to bring Caring Science into my facility. Each week I gained new skills and knowledge needed to become a Caritas Coach.

CREATING A CARING-HEALING ENVIRONMENT

Caring Science has helped to transform my cognitive-based mindset and change my nursing practice to one that is heart-centered and mindful. At the same time, creating transpersonal relationships with patients, coworkers, and leadership has helped to shift my work environment into a biogenic, compassionate, and caring-conscious field. In my Caritas Coach education I learned the value of being authentically present, honoring the talents of others, and respecting the energy that each person brings to the team. As a Caritas Coach, it is imperative that I continue to learn and grow while leading by example with loving-kindness to help create a caring-healing environment.

I use the 10 Caritas Processes as the foundation of my practice to help guide my consciousness; my ways of knowing; and my being, doing, and becoming. Each Caritas Process works with the others to develop a community of caring-healing relationships (Watson, 2008). By exhibiting loving-kindness toward self and others, I create a higher energy field. This helps sustain a healing environment. By being authentically present and open to the positive or negative emotions of others, and by using creative solution-finding skills in a caring manner, I can help sustain trusting and caring relationships.

ACTS OF SELF-CARE AND SELF-LOVE

When I start my day, I spend a moment breathing and meditating to center myself. I then set an intention for the day. This routine helps me to be authentically present with myself, which helps me become more self-aware and intentional with my actions. I encourage others to pause and center themselves, and I teach them different exercises to do this.

Each day I show loving-kindness to myself and others. I am mindful of the importance of self-care and self-love, which affects transpersonal relationships. If I am not in a good place within myself, I am not able to be authentic with others or show compassion. Acts of self-care and self-love that I practice include the following:

- Being mindful of how I think about myself and speak to myself

- Setting a positive intention every morning
- Thinking of one thing I am grateful for every day
- Stopping to enjoy the moment I am in
- Nourishing my body with healthy food and exercise
- Reminding myself that I am a priority

I also use meditation in my daily caring-healing practices. This practice affects me, and the environment around me, in a positive way. Using meditation, I can be still and quiet my mind, helping me to alleviate stress. I love to listen to the beautiful sounds of nature—the wind blowing through the trees, birds calling out to one another, ocean waves crashing onto the shore. Taking in each sound allows me to reflect on the little things for which I am grateful. The same is true for scents—like roses blooming or the fresh air after a spring rain shower—as well as listening to or playing music—this awareness can transport me to wherever I want to go in that moment.

On my nursing unit, one way I show loving-kindness to others is by offering anxious patients the opportunity to listen to therapeutic music using a CD player with headphones. I take slow breaths with the patient and then I offer the music. If they accept, I instruct them to close their eyes and think of a favorite place as they listen to the music. This calms the patient and has them smiling within minutes. We also play relaxing music throughout our unit via overhead speakers to create a healing environment for both staff and patients. The music is subtle but changes the energy in the room, helping each person to be calm and centered.

REFLECTING THROUGH JOURNALING AND POETRY

I use reflection to improve my practice. Reflection helps to relieve stress and bring me into a higher energetic field of caring. By reflecting on each situation and how I feel about it, I experience personal growth and gain a deeper and more fulfilling understanding of caritas literacy. I can then focus on what outcome I would have preferred in that moment and develop a plan to achieve that outcome the next time around. I also use reflection to develop awareness of my thoughts, feelings, and actions. Continuously reflecting and reviewing the 10 Caritas Processes reminds me how I can use loving-kindness to transform my community and myself.

Journaling is the practice of reflecting and putting your thoughts on paper. I use journaling in many ways. I write about good things that happened and reflect on how each positive experience transformed my thinking and energy level. I also write down experiences for which I am grateful and reflect on the many blessings that surround me. This helps to inform the way I show up each day. Journaling is a wonderful reflective practice. When I journal, I discover both my strengths and my weaknesses. I can then reflect on any changes I need to make in my practice. Or I can reflect on the changes I've already made and assess whether they helped me gain a deeper knowledge of self, others, or caritas literacy.

I also write poetry. I wrote the following poem during the CCEP as an aesthetic expression of personal knowing. It also illuminates how I create transpersonal moments with my patients. It reflects what I do with my patients in pre-op to help them think of a place that makes them happy and calms them down. It is an example of the transpersonal relationship between us.

While writing this poem, I thought of the many spirit-to-spirit connections I've made with patients while guiding them to visualize their favorite place. Listening to their stories has transported me all over the world. I have learned about their loved ones and the happy memories they have of them. The best part is seeing them relaxed, with eyes closed, and smiling.

I share some of these modalities with others so they can use them to create their own healing-caring practice. By helping others, I increase my energy and gain a sense of heart-centered wholeness.

OUR JOURNEY
By Heidi Hagle

Let's take a journey I say to you
Just listen to my voice and I'll talk you through
Your heart is racing, you are breathing so fast
Your body is so rigid, like it's encased in a cast
I place my hand on yours and pray
I feel your energy and want to take your fears away
I place a warm blanket to comfort you
A smile and a nod to show you I feel it too
Now tell me the one place you love to be
Close your eyes and I'll help you see
Take a deep breath then let it all go
Hear only my voice as if it is all that you know
Let's go on this journey together and see
A lasting moment in eternity

CHANGING THE ENERGETIC FIELD

When we give and receive love and kindness, we change the energetic field that surrounds us. Our spirit is lifted. We let go of ego-minded work and focus on heart-centered care.

Hope, kindness, faith, and gratitude all help us set our intentions and align with our spirit. When we set our intentions in positive ways, we lift our spirit and that of others. Our soul's purpose is to create spiritual and emotional growth. If we nurture our soul with positive affirmations and heart-centered care, we create a sense of well-being and happiness. If our soul is exposed to negative energy, we suffer. Setting our intention to express gratitude for self and other can create a space for trusting-caring relationships and cast our ego-mind to the side. When we make the connection and hold that heart-centered space, we connect with spirit and nurture our soul.

I use caritas literacy and the 10 Caritas Processes in my own Caritas Coach development. I allow each process to guide me with every person I encounter. Caritas literacy creates a learned set of ways of being that help me to bring a higher sense of self and care from my heart. It brings a caring consciousness into every relationship—with patients, coworkers, family, friends, and new acquaintances. I use authentic listening to be present and hear others' stories. This helps me see the whole person. I treat myself with loving-kindness. I treat others with loving-kindness and accept them for who they are. I encourage others while supporting their feelings. I care for their spirit to help uplift them.

Developing trusting-caring relationships means being aware of how I work with, communicate, and use Caring Science to promote open, caring, and constructive communication to disengage from negative biocidic behavior. Using caring-healing modalities and multiple ways of knowing—such as music, healing touch, breathing techniques, humor, laughter, and being open to unknown possibilities (Zander, 2007)—helps to create an environment of love and healing.

Caring moments also help to change the energy field. Some important caring acts that support the development of caring moments include the following:

- **Greeting everyone with a smile:** Smiling releases endorphins—chemicals in your brain that make you happy and reduce stress levels.

- **Acknowledging others for things they do:** Writing a brief handwritten note to express your thoughts or convey a simple thank you makes a big difference.

- **Giving authentic compliments to others:** Giving compliments uplifts the spirit and conveys loving-kindness and presence.

- **Setting an intention to listen:** Setting an intention to hear what the other is saying means you are fully present in the moment while showing compassion.

Mother Teresa once said, "Let us always meet each other with a smile, for the smile is the beginning of love" (Mother Teresa, 1979). This reminds me of the 10 Caritas Processes and is one of the caring-healing strategies I use each day.

CREATING A CARING COMMUNITY

We are all human. We may have moments when we are not present. But by creating a caring community, we can count on each other to help align us in spirit and work together in a higher energy field. If you are a Caritas Coach, others will look to you for guidance. They may not ask for it but they will watch how you practice caritas. If you experience a moment when you are not a healing presence, some may be quick to point this out. Still, by encouraging others to focus on heart-centered caring and ways of being, you can create a positive environment. This will help to build a community of people who lift each other up.

FINAL REFLECTIONS

Becoming a Caritas Coach has given me so many gifts to share with others. I have learned the value of self-love and creating caring moments. Through the CCEP I have gained the confidence to coach and to create a caring-healing environment for myself and others.

REFERENCES

Mother Teresa. (1979, December 11). Nobel lecture. Oslo, Norway.

Watson, J. (2008). *Nursing: The philosophy and science of caring* (rev. ed.). Boulder, CO: University Press of Colorado.

Zander, P. E. (2007). Ways of knowing in nursing: The historical evolution of a concept. *Journal of Theory Construction & Testing, 11*(1), 7–11.

RECONNECTION

–RACHEL JOHNSON-KOENKE, LCSW, CARITAS COACH

In this chapter, Rachel, a social worker in a healthcare setting, invites us to reconnect with who we are and what our purpose is through the framework of Caring Science. She shares how redefining her narrative from childhood has allowed her to focus on creating caring-healing relationships instead of simply completing the tasks of her life and work. Through the practices of centering, listening, empowerment, and acceptance, Rachel creates caring moments in which new chapters toward healing can begin.

RACHEL'S CARITAS JOURNEY

Being and becoming a Caritas Coach is a process of reconnecting with who you are and what your core purpose is, both professionally and personally. Like many social workers, I entered my profession because of a drive to help people by fostering deep and profound healing connections. I had endured trauma earlier in life, and a social worker had helped me to process it, redefine my story and myself, and find meaning in my experience. I saw myself as a survivor who could use my experience to help others who suffered similar trauma. I defined myself by my trauma and my victory over it.

As I progressed in my work as a social worker in a healthcare setting and in my own personal growth, I started questioning whether the narrative I held about my trauma was how I wanted to continue to define myself and my purpose. I had spent a large portion of my life identifying either as a victim of my trauma or as a survivor of my trauma. I knew I was more than that—that there was more that drove my purpose—but I felt unsure about how to frame my purpose and viewpoint of the world through a different lens than that of my traumatic experience.

LOVING SELF/LOVING OTHERS

Moving through the Caritas Coach Education Program (CCEP) enabled me to explore my life *before* my traumatic experience—before I started defining myself as either a victim or a survivor. As I worked through each of the Caritas Processes in the CCEP, I began to explore how to apply the same care and love to myself and my support systems that I provided for my clients. I started thinking about who I was before I defined myself by my trauma and how to reconnect with that version of myself. I began to repattern my thoughts and beliefs about the world and how I saw myself in it (Watson, 2008). I started to rewrite the story of who I was, what my purpose is, and what I wanted to become.

I realized that my love for all people—not my survival of a traumatic experience—drove my desire to help others. Although my traumatic experience gave me some of the skills I needed to help others, it was my deep love and care for others that drove my passion to help heal their pain and suffering.

One of my earliest memories is being at the grocery store as a small child, yelling "I love people!", hugging strangers, and telling them that I loved them. This profound love has always defined me. My work through the Caritas Processes allowed me to see how this love was also what drove my passion for helping people.

When someone else hurts, I hurt. This is not solely because of a sense of empathy for what the other person is going through, but because I hold the fundamental belief that we are all one and the same. When someone else hurts, I hurt—because we are all manifestations of the same universal field of caring and love (Watson, 2008). My passion for helping others springs from the realization of the deep spiritual connections between each of us. Thanks to the CCEP and my own personal growth, I now see these connections in a new and profound way.

AN INNER GLOW

As a child, I often noticed people around me who radiated love—how just being around them made others feel supported and cared for. They made those around them feel recharged and renewed. I called them "glowy people." More than anything I wanted to be like them. I had seen some of the darkness of the world but I wanted to radiate that glow of love for all beings. I wanted to be a part of the healing in the world.

I devoted myself to learning and growing as much as I could so I could nurture my own inner glow. I wanted to radiate healing and loving-kindness into the world and the multiverse. I pursued social work as a profession because I felt it would help me to cultivate this inner glow. Sometimes it did. I worked with one woman who had a long history of anxiety and suffered from shortness of breath. I was able to build a loving-healing relationship with her. This helped her to process her pain and past traumas and to explore the parts of her life that she was attempting to suppress—the parts where her anxiety was rooted. As a result, her anxiety decreased and her breathing improved.

But after working for a few years as a social worker in a healthcare setting, I found myself feeling frustrated with the limitations of the role. I knew the most helpful thing I could do was care about my clients. But as my caseload grew, I spent more and more of my workday performing tasks and completing forms—and documenting those tasks and forms. I had precious little time to sit with my clients—to truly be present with them. More and more, I felt a lack of connection with people in pain. This hampered my ability to transform their pain and suffering into love and true healing. I felt like my skills as a healthcare professional and healer were not being used.

I began to lose touch with the reason I had been drawn to social work in the first place. I looked to the literature to see if other social workers experienced similar struggles. What I found was a lack of definition of the role of social workers as healthcare professionals. Social workers focused less on building caring-healing relationships and more on completing paperwork and tasks (Craig & Muskat, 2013; Davidson, 1990). As my career moved into research, I became more interested in showing how social workers in a healthcare setting could do more than complete forms for people in need. They could be healing healthcare professionals.

TRANSPERSONAL CARING MOMENTS

Before my journey to becoming a Caritas Coach, I worked on a research study. My job on the study was to administer a structured social work intervention. During that same period, I went through a difficult and draining emotional time. I was able to go through the motions of the intervention but that was all I could manage. One day a participant in the intervention program expressed that he felt like no one listened to him. I paused to try to think of a response. My pause lasted too long, however. "Are you even listening?" he asked. He could feel my emotional disconnect—the lack of a transpersonal caring moment. After that, my rapport with the participant eroded. Although I tried to rebuild it, it was never quite the same. That experience taught me that there was so much more to the work I was doing then using the specific tools and techniques I had learned in school. I suddenly understood that I was growing a deeper connection with my clients and that it is from this deeper connection that healing springs.

Soon after, a colleague recommended that I read *Human Caring Science: A Theory of Nursing* by Dr. Jean Watson (2012). I was struck by the way the book encompassed so much of my life's pursuit to transform pain and suffering into love and healing. I was also struck by how much Caring Science aligned with and was complementary to the values and philosophies of social work. Dr. Watson's work introduced me to the notions of caring literacy and transpersonal caring moments.

I had felt transpersonal caring moments with clients. I had seen how these interactions had the power to reverberate into space-time, growing bigger than the moments themselves. I had often reflected on how, during these connected moments, I felt like I could actually make space for my clients' healing. But I had only experienced these caring moments when they occurred naturally. I knew there was something going on in these moments—something I hadn't been able to articulate. I believed I made a difference in their healing because I truly cared. But I couldn't figure out how or why this occurred until I read Dr. Watson's book. I had not realized there was a way to cultivate and create space for these moments. It wasn't until I became more caring literate (Watson, 2008) that I understood what these moments were and how to create space for them to grow and expand. Watson writes:

> The caring moment can be an existential turn-
> ing point for the nurse, in that it involves pausing,
> choosing to "see"; it is informed action guided by an
> intentionality and consciousness of how to be in the
> moment—fully present, open to the other person,
> open to compassion and connection, beyond the
> ego-control focus that is so common. (2008, p. 5)

When I saw that these moments could be created, I began to understand how to make space for my clients to heal themselves. One method was to center myself before meeting with each client. I envisioned caring and healing energy surrounding me. Then as I met with the client, I imagined wrapping him or her in the energy I generated.

I tried this with one client who was struggling to accept the difficulties imposed on him by heart failure. Having centered myself before our telephone session, I encouraged him to begin the process of accepting his limitations. "If I accept these limitations it means I'm giving up!" the man cried. "I can't do that!" He began to weep and then hung up on me. Afterward I questioned whether pushing him had been the right thing to do. I got my answer a week or so later when the client called me back. First he apologized for hanging up so abruptly. Then he told me he had realized he *could* accept his limitations. He could redefine who he was and what was truly important to him. He could rewrite his story. He said our conversation had not just changed his perception of how his illness had affected him; it had changed his life.

In my social work education and clinical experience, I have been taught many important lessons. I've been taught the value of empowering people to make changes for themselves. I've been taught to trust that clients are the experts in their own lives. I've been taught to meet people where they are, not where I (or the system in which I work) want them to be. I've been taught to believe in the possibilities for growth and change. Finally, I've been taught to honor the sacredness of each person's story. When these values live at the center of social work practice, it can make a dramatic difference in each individual's quality of life and even encourage the process of healing.

I have always believed people exist as a "living, growing gestalt" (Watson, 2012, p. 66)—that is, surrounded by, while being part of, the systems in which they reside. My clinical experience as a social worker deepened my understanding of the interconnectedness of all living beings and helped me grasp on a profound level the importance of connections and relationships as we work to improve people's lives. But the process of being and becoming a Caritas Coach has shown me how Caring Science nurtures the caring-loving connections and transpersonal caring moments that are the building blocks of all relationships and systems.

Caring-Loving Connections

Through the CCEP, I learned caring literacy (Watson, 2008)—a language to describe caring moments and the love and healing that take place in transpersonal relationships. I also found a community of people who understand these aspects of caring, love, and healing. I discovered that Caring Science not only encompassed my own personal spiritual belief system—a system I had held since childhood—but also represented the root of my passion for transforming the healthcare social work profession by reconnecting it with true caring and healing. I realized this passion could spur me to redefine the role of healthcare social work and even to redefine health and the healthcare system itself.

By working through the 10 Caritas Processes as part of my caritas journey, I learned how to grow transpersonal caring moments into my clinical practice and how to create the space to allow for transpersonal caring (Watson, 2008). I began to refocus the purpose of my clinical work to nurture these transpersonal caring moments. These moments are now the bedrock of my clinical social work practice—the foundation of all the other techniques I use. If I am not present or do not practice loving-kindness *or* accept both the negative and positive feelings of my clients and myself, then the clinical techniques I use won't have the same effect.

The foundation of my work is reconnecting with caring and loving energy and relationships by building transpersonal caring moments with everyone around me—not just clients, but coworkers, friends, and family. I strive to start each day by centering myself so that I can be prepared for each interaction. I envision a transfer of energy between me and my clients, my coworkers, and my family and friends that lifts all of us up to a place of healing.

Transpersonal caring and healing are the basis of my clinical practice and research. It drives my relationships with all the systems that surround me. This "transpersonal perspective allows us to go beyond physical-ego self to the quiet depths of the soul...[to] connect with that which is timeless and eternal" (Watson, 2012, p. 58). This connection to the depths of my soul nurtures my healing inner glow that then radiates into the multiverse. By tapping into that transpersonal connection with the wholeness of the multiverse, the transpersonal caring-healing moment is both life-giving and life-receiving—a full and complete circle. The transpersonal caring moment exists outside of space-time. "Past, present, and future instants merge and fuse" (Watson, 2012, p. 72), radiating out into the multiverse. This moment becomes "part of the subjective, lived reality, and the life history of both (nurse and patient)" (Watson, 2012, p. 73). The transpersonal caring moment affects all the systems and connections between each of us.

The love at the center of the transpersonal caring moment is the core of who I am and who I want to be. Love is the purpose of my life. It is the focus of my work with my clients and of my growth as a person and social work researcher. Love is the basis for the transformation from pain and suffering to healing through the Caritas

Processes (Watson, 2008). Without love for my clients, my profession, healthcare systems, and myself, it is difficult, if not impossible, to achieve healing or find meaning.

FINAL REFLECTIONS

From new insights gained through my personal caritas journey and experiences as a Caritas Coach, I recognize that my purpose is to expand my personal inner glow so that it reaches healthcare systems and the professions of healthcare social work and nursing. By helping to define the role of social workers in healthcare systems as professional healers who help people to write (and in some cases, rewrite) the stories of their life experiences, I can nurture that glow so that it radiates into the future of healthcare and touches the lives of countless beings. My Caritas Coach journey has been a glowing circle connecting me to who I was, who I am, and who I will become.

REFERENCES

Craig, S. L., & Muskat, B. (2013). Bouncers, brokers, and glue: The self-described roles of social workers in urban hospitals. *Health & Social Work, 38*(1), 7–16.

Davidson, K. W. (1990). Role blurring and the hospital social worker's search for a clear domain. *Health & Social Work, 15*(3), 228–234.

Watson, J. (2008). *Nursing: The philosophy and science of caring* (rev. ed.). Boulder, CO: University Press of Colorado.

Watson, J. (2012). *Human caring science: A theory of nursing* (2nd ed.). Burlington, MA: Jones & Bartlett Learning.

.

The Learning Path of a Caritas Coach Nurse

–Diane Poulios, MA, RN, CHCR, AHN-BC, Caritas Coach

In this chapter, Diane invites us to explore caritas literacies. These serve as a guide to seeing self, others, and the world as whole, valued, and interconnected. Emphasizing all ways of knowing, Diane explores how integrating this approach into her interviewing practices and hiring decisions helps to ensure a good fit for the organization. Finally, Diane shares her experiences incorporating a spiritual dimension into her caring-healing practice. This adds an element of the sacred to the purpose, intentions, and actions of the Caritas Coach and serves as a professional development guide for all healthcare professionals.

DIANE'S CARITAS JOURNEY

For me, the key part of the question, "What does it mean to be and become a Caritas Coach?" is not the label "Caritas Coach," but the words *be* and *become*. Being and becoming define the dynamic ongoing process of Caring Science.

One does not merely study Caring Science, learn its principles and dimensions, and suddenly possess the ability to manifest competency as a Caritas Coach. The evolution of a Caritas Coach is not linear. Rather, it is an inward journey of winding roads that lead to new ways of thinking, feeling, and becoming. The journey invites an exploration of previously held ideas about self and the world. These ideas are figuratively tossed up into the universe and allowed to float back down and realign, enabling us to reinterpret our beliefs and stories through new eyes and wisdom. In this way we become a slowly transformed and transforming spirit.

As we integrate this knowledge with our spirituality and beliefs about self, the world, and our higher power, this caring-loving energy finds a home in our heart. So as we live Caring Science, it creates a foundation of meaning and living—framed in pan-dimensional time, language, creativity, and love—that reflects a new life, spirit, and philosophy, and a renewed relationship with the world. As Watson writes, "Caring and love ultimately become one...we are all called to care, and it is through the energy of Love that we reach out to the universe of possibilities to connect with Other, nature and that which is greater and more magnificent than our isolated separate, physical-ego existence alone" (Watson, 2005, p. 54).

Of course this is not to say the transition is easy. We struggle with previously held beliefs. This new way of being and becoming is organically tested, challenged, and sometimes masked as we enter each helical turn of change, growth, and understanding. Rogers defines the world as manifesting a helical pattern of increasing complexity and diversity of energetic frequencies. As the helix turns there is a downward spiral that is inherent in the process of transformation (Rogers, 1988). This explains the meaning of being and becoming.

Transformation is a process of stepping back, letting go, acknowledging self, and eventually moving forward with the new. There is often conflict before transformation. Internal turmoil ensues when we pause to challenge and make sense of new ways of thought. This all occurs before the backdrop of the universe itself, which—seen or unseen—is changing as well. Chaos and conflict come before clarity and unity. Anguish comes before joy.

Being and becoming is the dynamic nature of life and part of what it means to be human. The universe has given us the gift of being conscious of this process, especially if we allow ourselves to be active rather than passive as we journey through it. My ninth grade English teacher challenged the class to write without using the verb "to be" in any form due to what he felt was its inactive and passive nature. He believed there were more descriptive and powerful verbs. Upon reflection as I have undergone the process of being and becoming, I wish he would have allowed responsive discourse regarding this statement. He could have dedicated time to discussing the dynamic nature, power, and use of the verb "to be" in all its conjugations. *Being* can have great meaning.

As a Caritas Coach I am introduced to ways of thinking and being, as well as to practices and methods that are considered unconventional in the Western world. For example, Westerners learn of Newton's third law of motion, which states that for every action (or change) there is an equal and opposite reaction (Newton, 1687). This universal phenomenon is evident and organic. In contrast, a Caritas Coach influences self, others, and the world by integrating and preserving space to allow for a different kind of process not beholden to conventional paradigms. We do this by identifying with another person's story, synchronizing with one's life story, and withholding judgment. We help draw connections, identify patterns, create resonance, and guide one toward emergent readiness. In other words, a Caritas Coach encourages new ways of thinking within the Newtonian law of time and action-reaction. The coach faithfully trusts that in this process, a higher good unfolds. The inherent nature of this process is dynamic, emergent, and without hierarchal force (Watson, 2005). When one resonates with this unique caring way of perceiving the world, one is less inclined to revert to the conventional pure Newtonian way of thinking and being.

HEALING HUMANITY WITH UNIVERSAL COMPASSION

I have always felt a strong connection to God or a higher divine force that allows us to surrender to its goodness and love. This inspirational and loving energy spoke forcefully to my heart and soul, calling me to nursing as a child. I understood from a young age that I was meant to serve and care for others. My soul was drawn to a universal compassion for humanity.

As a graduate nursing student, I became interested in the science of unitary human beings, a nursing worldview espoused by Dr. Martha Rogers. This worldview is an integral part of Watson's science of human caring. This led me to study complementary healing arts such as therapeutic touch, craniosacral therapy, reflexology, shiatsu, creative visualization, and the relaxation response.

I began using these modalities to help cancer patients in hospitals. One was a young female colon cancer patient who was experiencing great pain and anxiety after surgery. I described to her the healing effects of therapeutic touch and asked if she'd like me to administer it to her. She agreed to receive the treatment. After 10 minutes of treatment, the patient smiled. She was amazed by her experience during the treatment. She told me that during the treatment she saw colors and felt a much-needed sense of healing peace. Interestingly I had seen the same colors. We also shared a sense of time as pan-dimensional. Although the treatment lasted only 10 minutes, we both felt we had experienced a healing moment that was much longer.

In contrast, I once cared for a young female patient who had been surgically dismembered during treatment for sarcoma (with little attention to her spirit). This was years before I studied Caring Science. It seemed that during her entire hospital stay, she simply lay in her bed and cried. Her suffering was so extreme, no one quite knew how to *be* with her. Years later, after I had studied Caring Science, and a philosophy of healing and practice of unconditional love had crystalized in my mind, I wondered how healing that patient's experience could have been if she'd had a caritas nurse alongside her!

Whether at the point of care, while teaching, or while recruiting staff, Caring Science provides a foundation to actualize true nursing. The theory is clear, foundational, dynamic, focused, and ever evolving to include new ways of knowing and understanding humanity and the world. Nurses help others make sense of critical experiences in ways other professionals may not. Healing humanity is at the core of nursing. Now more than ever, Caring Science illuminates the true essence of nursing and provides the best home in which the nursing spirit and heart can dwell. "It is life giving and life receiving" (Watson, 2008, p. 58).

CREATING AN ATMOSPHERE OF OPENNESS AND HONESTY

I work as a nurse recruiter. As part of my job I interview candidates for placement. The purpose of any job interview is to provide the candidate with an opportunity to research the hiring organization and to enable the interviewer or recruiter to assess whether the candidate is the right fit for the organization (and vice versa). Whether someone is the right fit depends on whether he or she resonates with the organization on a mental, moral, and clinical level. Various factors come into play, such as skill set, accountability, leadership abilities, values, personality, energy, culture, and beliefs about nursing practice.

Naturally, candidates often feel nervous or unsure when they enter the interview room. This can jeapordize open communication. To combat this I have taken several steps. One is to create a relaxed environment. Our environment and the living entities within it can be defined in terms of energy and energy waves. Huismann,

Morales, Van Hoof, and Kort (2012) show that the intentional use of color, nature, and aromas can influence this energy, as they all translate into healing frequencies. With this evidence in mind, we painted the interview room a soft green—the color of life, renewal, and groundedness—and hung images of ocean scenes on the wall. We also infuse the room with a relaxing lavender aroma. Finally, the room contains figurines that relate to nursing or to universal kindness and caring, including one of Florence Nightingale. Simply put, our environment affects how we feel and therefore how we communicate. The more relaxed the environment, the more open candidates feel to communicate their true selves (Chesser, 2017).

My own energy also affects each interview. I'm a sentient and pan-dimensional being. Therefore, I am an integral part of my environment and those around me (Rogers, 1970). As a Caritas Coach, I am obligated to use Caring Science in all my interactions—including interviews. That means exhibiting both transpersonal caring and *transpersonal presence*. Transpersonal caring is the transformational integration of caring energies between living entities with an intention to help or to heal. It "invites full loving kindness and equanimity of presence of another...that can be a turning point in one's life" for all entities involved (Watson, 2008, p. 79). To possess transpersonal presence, one must first be intentionally present with self.

To achieve this—and to shift the field toward wholeness, goodwill, and healing—I begin each day with a meditative prayer. This helps me to center myself so I can create caring relationships with others while feeling loved and cared for. I hold a positive intention to smile at others and show kindness to all with whom I interact. I also take deep breaths to center myself before an interview. Research shows that mindful breathing establishes a synchronicity in the body between the sympathetic and parasympathetic systems, resulting in calm and focus (Benson & Proctor, 2010). Finally, I greet candidates with a warm smile. I welcome them by saying, "It's an honor to meet you" and by offering water, almost as a blessing. Manifesting transpersonal caring brings down barriers and creates an atmosphere of open and honest dialogue and transformation.

During the interview itself, I use all ways of knowing. Our interview questionnaire and evaluation form are rooted in Watson's science of human caring and the 10 Caritas Processes. For example, we ask the candidate to "describe the experience(s) in your life that has affected the way in which you view humanity or has influenced your reason for being in this world." This question often takes candidates by surprise. However, they do not hesitate to share their stories in response. One candidate explained that her father died in her arms, and she believed she could "speak" to him every day by becoming a nurse. Another question asks candidates to describe someone in their profession they admire and the impact that person has had on their life and development. When asked, this question evokes feelings of gratitude and honor. The interview questions are open-ended to encourage self-reflection and to help to reveal each candidate's higher self. Patterns, commonalities, and transformational experiences often unfold. This transpersonal process, made possible by authentic communication and caring literacy, enhances my ability to determine a good fit—or a resonance between the energies of the candidate and that of the organization. Interestingly, the limited 30-minute interview time frame often seems to expand and contract in response to the ebb and flow of the interview.

CARING LITERACY: A GUIDE TO PROFESSIONAL DEVELOPMENT

One cannot manifest transpersonal caring without calling on caring literacy. Caring literacy is how we put Caring Science into action.

I live and breathe Caring Science. It is who I am. I progress from living in the world to witnessing it, experiencing it, and understanding it, as I become more fully myself—a self that is constantly evolving, just like the world around me. I don't think of it as constantly chasing myself as I strive for progress—rather, I feel as if

I am enveloping myself in acceptance and love, which encourages further becoming. Caring literacy integrates an evolving emotional intelligence, consciousness, intentionality, sensitivity, and efficacy that cultivate skills and awareness of loving-kindness integral to one's professional being (Watson, 2008). Through caring literacy, I have been able to express my soul and spirit to all I encounter. How I present myself is a direct reflection of my relationship to the world. If Caring Science is my spiritual essence, then I can be beautiful, and so can the world and people around me.

I use caring literacy as a guide for my professional development. Indeed, my quest for caring literacy has fused with an interest in holistic health coaching. In addition to becoming a Caritas Coach, I have also become a certified holistic health coach. This provides me with another way to offer one-on-one or group healing and love to others. Caring Science works as a backdrop to interpret the holistic health program, while caring literacy provides me with an implementation method—a way to practice Caring Science in various facets of my work and my life.

I also work with others to provide caring-healing classes to nurses throughout our system. These 1-day classes cover holistic nursing, self-care, and the importance of viewing the world and our patients through the lens of Caring Science. Through the class we reawaken our nurses to why they went into nursing, as well as the importance of their roles and influences in the world. Most importantly, these classes introduce the concept of transpersonal caring and loving presence. It is a powerful program for self-care and affirmation. Helping to create, develop, and present this program has been a great expression of my own love for the nursing profession. I'm proud that our nursing leadership understands how important this is and desires to help our nurses feel valued and cared for!

PERSONAL DISCOVERY OF BEAUTY AND UNIVERSAL LOVE

Self-reflection and self-awareness do not always come easily. Critiquing oneself takes courage and skill. Often it is painful. But intentionally opening ourselves to greater awareness is both enriching and transformational.

As a young teen, I spent one summer away from my family while working on a ranch in Colorado. I didn't know anyone else there, nor was there anyone else my age. Although I was excited about being away, I missed my family. To ease my yearning for their presence, I took frequent walks in the mountains. Through self-reflection during these walks I realized how dear my parents were to me and how lucky I was to be their daughter. I also witnessed the magnificent beauty of our world. I felt a oneness with God or spirit that was beyond articulation. I felt soothed by my abundant thoughts of gratitude and the nature that lovingly embraced me. The warm wind against my cheeks and the blue-purple sky were sacred to me.

I began to look forward to my daily sacred walks of prayer and comforting beauty. Nature offered me strength and purpose as I performed my housekeeping chores at the ranch. This experience made me feel at one with the universe, and my spirit soared to places it had never been before. Although I felt like a small being in the midst of grandeur, I did not feel insignificant. I was part of a living entity that needed me as much as I needed it in order to be whole. What I felt, I realized, was love. "Such becomingness makes sense within a pan-dimensional framework of unfolding patterns in human time" (Poulios, 1997, p. 230).

I returned home wiser and calmer. I felt sustained. My experience had a harmonious lingering presence. This transcendental feeling of love stayed with me through college, on my wedding day, at my first job, and when I gave birth. It was a gift. It nourished me and those around me on my life journey. It only takes one person to change the energy of a room, and it only takes one person to shift how others experience the world toward love and harmony. These miracles in life that seem small have far greater influence than our awareness permits.

We can draw on these moments of peace and love at will. The divine engages, loves, and comforts upon request through prayer and meditation. Sometimes a feeling of divine energy comes without warning through the transcending language of music or nature. Through self-reflection and the awareness of being connected with the divine, I have faith that I will always be comforted and guided through life.

FINAL REFLECTIONS

My journey as a Caritas Coach started when I discovered my path to nursing as a young girl. Learning about Caring Science, experiencing healing moments of lingering presence, and realizing that love and caring are organically symbiotic requires a shift from a closed way of thinking to one that is open and accepting. As we dwell in this space, we become embodied by a way of living, being, and becoming that reflects peace and connection with a greater good. My path reflects the wonder, experiences, and challenges of illuminating the life of a caritas nurse. It is not a point in time but a flowing existence of constant unfolding along a path of caring for humanity, self, and the world. I embrace and wonder at this path every day. "Today, open your mind, your heart, and your life to that which you don't yet know, that you might contain that which is greater than yourself" (Cahn, 2016, p. 1).

REFERENCES

Benson, H., & Proctor, W. (2010). *Relaxation revolution: The science and genetics of mind body healing.* New York, NY: Scribner.

Cahn, J. (2016). *The book of mysteries.* Lake Mary, FL: Frontline.

Chesser, J. (2017). *Human resources management in a hospitality environment.* Boca Raton, FL: CRC Press.

Huisman, E. R. C. M., Morales, E., Van Hoof, J., & Kort, H. S. M. (December 2012). Healing environment: A review of the impact of physical environmental factors on users. *Building and Environment, 58,* 70–80.

Newton, I. (1687). *Philosophiæ naturalis principia mathematica (mathematical principles of natural philosophy).* London, UK: Imprimature Press.

Poulios, D. A. (1997). A celebration of unitary human beings: Becoming a mother. In M. Madrid (Ed.), *Patterns of Rogerian knowing* (p. 230). New York, NY: National League for Nursing Press.

Rogers, M. E. (1970). *An introduction to the theoretical basis of nursing.* Philadelphia, PA: F. A. Davis Co.

Rogers, M. E. (1988). Nursing science and art: A prospective. *Nursing Science Quarterly, 1*(3), 99–102.

Watson, J. (2005). *Caring science as sacred science.* Philadelphia, PA: F. A. Davis Co.

Watson, J. (2008). *Nursing: The philosophy and science of caring* (rev. ed.). Boulder, CO: University Press of Colorado.

5

CARITAS LEADERSHIP: MODELING HEART-CENTERED PRAXIS

TRANSFORMATION THROUGH CARING MOMENTS

–STEPHANIE AHMED, DNP, FNP-BC, DPNAP, CARITAS COACH

Stephanie shares how she fosters an environment that supports the development of an organizational culture in which nurses are encouraged to practice from a Caring Science framework. Like others have described in this text, she demonstrates how this process begins with her own commitment to engage in a personal caritas journey and how this serves as a foundation for relating to others. Stephanie provides examples of how Caring Science is threaded throughout her department, including job descriptions, model of care, employment practices, and performance review. She uses the distinctive opportunity she has as a nursing director to influence caritas literacy throughout her organization.

STEPHANIE'S CARITAS JOURNEY

In *Nursing: The Philosophy and Science of Caring* (2008), Watson speaks conceptually of the nurse whose professional practice arises from an evolved form of consciousness—one which serves to connect the nurse to the humanity of self and others. Engaging from a heart-centered framework, the nurse operationalizes the Caritas Processes, and through this relational way of being, actively becomes an extension of the caring-healing environment. Within the context of human caring theory (HCT), the human connection is recognized to be equally as important for the nurse as it is for the patient. When optimal, this connection is described as biogenic, life-giving, and life-sustaining (Watson, 2008).

Practicing as a nursing director and a Caritas Coach, I have the opportunity to create an environment and influence organizational culture that supports nurses to practice from an HCT framework. Foundational to that work is the development of job descriptions and performance measures, which reflect the organization's professional practice model and commitment to developing a nursing workforce that practices using a Caring Science foundation.

CREATING A CARITAS ORGANIZATIONAL CULTURE

Creating an organizational caritas culture begins with a process of developing a shared awareness for HCT. Strategies used to disseminate caring literacy to others have included development and co-facilitation of an educational program for nursing directors and nurse educators related to HCT core concepts and practices, and creation of an HCT toolbox of resources designed to assist nursing directors in rapidly incorporating HCT practices among staff and promoting reflective practice. The toolbox included narratives framed around ambulatory practice and Haldorsdottir's model (Watson, 2008, p. 26) and a library of 30 days of caritas intentions corresponding to the Caritas Processes.

With an intention to impact the patient care experience in the primary care practices, nurses (both RNs and LPNs) across the organization's 14 practices and 2 health centers were led in a half-day retreat that focused largely on HCT core concepts and practices. To promote reflective practice and "giving language" to the work of caring, a narrative was read describing an ambulatory team-based care encounter between a nurse and patient. Participants were asked to discuss and apply Haldorsdottir's model, reflecting on the *ways of being* incorporated into the narrative. Through this exercise, nurses were encouraged to develop a heightened awareness of those caring behaviors considered biogenic and life-sustaining.

Reflective practice skills have been developed through leading and participating in a twice-weekly Touchstones group meetings with nursing leadership. Started by the Chief Nursing Officer (CNO), also a Caritas Coach, Touchstones provided a sense of community and an opportunity to engage in a centering exercise that promotes setting an intention and consciousness for caring and healing (Watson, 2008). The group used a singing bowl to call the circle and practiced heart-centered breathing exercises while promoting an environment with caring intention. Centering is foundational to a practice of loving-kindness, enabling a focus on and commitment to caring, and further facilitates operationalizing the Caritas Processes. Through regular Touchstones participation, I began to notice that my relationship with the CNO, members of the nurse executive board, and nursing director peers began to deepen. A sense of connection grew beyond the participants of Touchstones to include the institution—and thus, importantly, to the staff.

As I became aware of my own transformation through Touchstones, I wanted to share the experience with nursing staff and others in the hopes of facilitating their own caritas journeys. I sought opportunities to open committee and staff meetings with the setting of a caring intention and the use of a singing bowl. The singing bowl was initially received with curiosity, but by sharing my own personal experience with it and using a little bit of humor, staff became more comfortable and willing to give it a try. I was able to create an openness by acknowledging the bowl was unusual at first for me too. I explained that over time I recognized a Pavlovian response. While Pavlov's dogs equated the sound of the bell with food, my mind equated the sound of the singing bowl with the positive experiences I had in the Touchstones group; it gave me permission to relax, center, and think. I described how I could feel the vibration of the bowl before it actually became audible to others and used this as a metaphor to illustrate our own vibration as we engaged in caring and healing. I asked the staff questions such as:

- What vibe do you give off when you enter the exam room?

- Are you in a hurry or do you connect to the patient in a caring way—maybe a kind touch, a hand on the shoulder? (There are so many ways we can "touch" people.)

- What does it look like when you put the blood pressure cuff on the first patient of the day? What does it look like when you put the blood pressure cuff on the last patient of the day?

- Are we seeking those opportunities to connect and to touch? Or as we get busy, are we paying attention more to the tasks and not to the person who needs our care?

Instantly they got it, and so did I—I became awakened that I too have so many ways (directly and indirectly) to touch patients and staff through modeling a caring consciousness! Soon requests came for me to attend staff meetings and I was advised to "bring the bowl." The staff was appreciative of this new and interesting multisensory experience.

Because nursing leadership recognized that from the front desk to the exam room everyone is an extension of our organization's caring and healing environment, HCT content has been shared with physicians, social workers, practice managers, medical assistants, front desk staff, human resource personnel, and even organization VPs. In this way, an invitation has been extended broadly, encouraging and nurturing the development of an organizational network that connects very intentionally with caring and humanity—that of self and other.

NURSE RECRUITMENT GOVERNED BY THE HUMAN CARING THEORY FRAMEWORK

As nursing director and caritas leader, there is a responsibility to uphold the professional practice model (PPM) of the organization. The PPM expresses a commitment to nurses as authentic leaders and supports such values as shared decision-making, relationship-based care, nursing scholarship, outcome-focused measures, and diversity and inclusivity. This model of nursing practice is underpinned by HCT. As we strive to create congruence between stated values and nursing roles, the use of HCT creates a deliberate space for the carative work of nurses in the job description, expressing expectations of a humanized model of care. Logically, it also influences aspects of leadership, including interviews conducted during the hiring process and subsequent performance reviews.

The healthcare environment is rapidly changing, and care redesign has become a major organizational focus. Anticipating an evolution in nursing roles that will utilize registered nurses in our organization's well-established primary care teams, language that supports practicing from an HCT-informed framework has been incorporated into the newly developed job description. Care delivery models of the future will increasingly rely on nurses to successfully coordinate complex care and to support and coach patients with chronic disease toward mutually shared goals. The human caring theory offers the foundation upon which helping-trusting-caring relationships can be developed between nurses and patients. Engaging patients in the context of a transpersonal caring relationship, a caritas-informed nurse understands the need to remain within the frame of reference of the patient. The nurse is naturally attuned to and engaged with the patient and possesses the ability to "read the field," interpreting those verbal and nonverbal cues that dynamically evolve, impacting care delivery outcomes. This relational expertise, more appropriately stated as caring literacy, is necessary for professional nursing to "make connections between caring and healing/

health/wholeness outcomes, transcending conventional outcomes of curing alone" (Watson, 2008, p. 79). As organizations are held accountable to the metrics of value-driven care, and the outcomes of such care are publicly reported, nurses practicing from an HCT framework have the potential to positively influence the patient care experience and the reported data. Further, as competition in the healthcare market increases, ensuring patients a healing, transpersonal experience is a way not only to attract new patients but also to enhance the organization's ability to attract and retain the best nurses!

While the job description describes the role, practice setting, and qualifications required for a specific position, the interview process enables an evaluation of an applicant's job-related skills. Behavioral-based interviewing techniques are commonly employed and thought to be predictive of the applicant's capabilities. However, this form of interviewing is typically not used to support an assessment of embodied caritas attributes. To enhance my practice using a caritas way of being, I adapted my interviewing style to better elicit those values expressed in a transpersonal caring-consciousness relationship. I explored this with the applicants by asking them to share a caring moment exemplar from their own professional practice and discussing it with them. The interview is conceptually framed within the context of the organization's professional practice model and selection of Watson's human caring theory to underpin the caring practice of nursing. Applicants are reassured that the interview is not a test, but rather an opportunity for bidirectional sharing. Through the interview process, they are able to get to know and understand the values of the nursing department. It is also a means by which they can share their own values and experiences as a nurse. The applicant is provided with a copy of the Caritas Processes and a brief description of HCT and asked to review it. Upon completion, the applicant then has an opportunity to share initial impressions of the Caritas Processes. Frequently, applicants make statements such as, "This is how I want to practice," or, "This is how I wish I could practice." While simply the indication of HCT appeal or lack thereof is not considered predictive, discussions based on the applicants' own practice exemplars do provide a window of understanding into their experiences of developing loving and trusting relationships and supporting the faith, hope, and belief system of others, and can even be an indication of how the applicant might give and receive both positive and negative feedback.

It has been most common for applicants to speak about developing and sustaining helping-trusting-caring relationships; however, a recent interview with an advanced practice nurse was notable because she chose to speak about Caritas Process 5—being present to and supportive of the expression of positive and negative feelings. She connected that Caritas Process to an incident in which she prescribed a medication at a dose that was higher than recommended for a pediatric patient. Although the error was relatively benign and most likely would never have been detected, the applicant detailed her immediate engagement of the patient's parents by both informing them and apologizing. She described how she notified management and completed the required safety documentation of the error. She spoke of the impact the error had on her confidence as a provider and how she was able to subsequently move forward. Telling the story of a medication error during an interview was courageous, and attributes of caring consciousness were evident throughout the discussion. In acknowledging the error, and through her detailed response to it, the applicant demonstrated that she was both human and humane. Her actions supported recognition of the intrinsic worth of the vulnerable pediatric patient who was unable to advocate for self, and her recognized responsibility to be that patient's advocate without regard to risk of self. While acknowledging the medication error, the applicant described a way of being that was truly biogenic, life-sustaining, and supported a level of caring consciousness that placed the best interests of the patient first. Discussion of the exemplar further revealed much about her ethics, integrity, and professional values, which might not have been evident through other interviewing styles. Structuring the interviews around the Caring Processes and the caring moment provides an opportunity to know the applicant more deeply. It also allows me to be strategic about hiring those individuals who not only possess the necessary technical skills but also demonstrate a greater potential to have the relational, caring attributes that are requisite of caring consciousness.

THE ANNUAL REVIEW GROUNDED IN CARING SCIENCE

Nurses are called to care, and while Watson describes an evolved being/ontological presence that is required for professionals engaged in caring and healing, the practice of nursing has historically been assessed in alignment with role-related tasks and outcomes. With the recent training of primary care nursing staff in HCT, including the incorporation of HCT as part of the RN job description, annual performance appraisals are positioned to be framed around Caring Science and the professional practice model. My own growth and development as a caritas-informed nursing leader is assisting me to transform the annual review, previously perceived as a perfunctory human resource requirement, into an opportunity for deeper engagement with the caring practices of nurses. Similar to the interview process, by focusing on caring moments as a means of reflective practice I am fostering a greater understanding of how primary care registered nurses demonstrate caring literacy. Frequently, primary care nurses engage patients telephonically, or electronically via email. The lack of physical proximity between the patient and the nurse has the potential to create challenges with reading the field and successful engagement. Interesting questions to explore might include:

- How does the nurse read the field when engaging telephonically?

- How is authentic presence established?

- How is authentic listening different in person than on the telephone?

- How does the nurse convey his/her authenticity and unconditional loving-kindness when engaging by phone or email with a patient?

In a recent discussion with an experienced triage nurse, I remarked about her skill to "transcend the telephone" and create meaningful connections with patients. I asked what she thought contributed to her success. She reported that when engaging telephonically with patients, she always recalls a specific and particularly meaningful patient interaction that occurred many years earlier. In asking her what she remembered about the encounter, she said, "So many years later, I still remember his name today," and, "in thinking about him, I am able to reconnect with the caring in me." She reported that the encounter was "mutually fulfilling"—it met the patient's need for help, but also fulfilled her own need to help the patient. In her current practice of telephone triage, she mentally revisits that positive experience over and over. It is her "gold standard" and guides her daily interactions with patients. This transformative experience provided us with the opportunity to conceptually frame caring as not constrained by time or space. Together we reflected on how she was changed by the interaction and how it informed subsequent patient encounters. We discussed authentic presence, deep listening, and use of verbal cues to convey engagement and understanding. Nurses are required to engage in lifelong learning. As a nursing director, it would be easy to view this requirement through a limited lens, attributing the need to learn merely as an academic task-based experience. However, as a Caritas Coach, I recognize that Watson is calling us toward a deeper process of learning and development through a continually evolving emotional heart intelligence and consciousness. Caring moment discussions present an opportunity for me to nurture the nurse's understanding of HCT and encourage the self-growth and awareness that is necessary to cultivate caritas consciousness.

Watson (2008) suggests that those caring attributes, recognized as both human and humane, can be developed with intentionality. Occurring in the context of a conscious evolution, such development entails expanding one's heart-centered intelligence and emotional skill set, opening to a higher-level, energetic, and infinite spiritual field of one's humanity (Watson, 2008). It is an awakening of spirit that generates a reverence for the humanity of self and other, but further, expands the understanding of these concepts in relation to the broader world. Self-perception, cultivated since birth as *individual* now shifts, and a strong sense of connectivity to others, and to the world, begins to emerge. This evolution in thinking and relational way of being has the potential to transform nursing and the anticipated impacts of the discipline and its roles. As nursing director, becoming a Caritas Coach has transformed my thinking and way of being with respect to my role and the ambulatory setting in which I practice. As a leader and member of a discipline that has a responsibility for moral action, I am bound to "give voice" on behalf of others.

Transforming Nursing Leadership: A New Perspective

My responsibilities as the ambulatory nursing director include the provision of operational support for nursing practice across a variety of primary care, medical, and surgical specialty clinics. I establish standards for clinical practice, develop job descriptions, evaluate nursing practice, and develop related policies to support the work of the nurses. Management of staff is implicit to this role, and related duties range from clinical coaching and mentorship, to acting as confidant, to participating in crucial conversations that address accountability and expectations, and at times, termination. The Caritas Processes provide an operational framework for a leadership practice of loving-kindness and equanimity and serves as a compass to establish a transpersonal presence. As I continue to incorporate an HCT framework into my practice, I've noticed my leadership style has become less hierarchical, with a decided shift towards servant leadership—acting in service to the patients, the staff, and the organization. I do not need to manage; rather, I teach, coach, and encourage. I *love*.

Leading is achieved most frequently from influence and persuasion, thus a culture for participatory decision-making is created. Staff report feeling supported and highly engaged, and team relationships have deepened. I have developed an appreciation for learning to modulate my own energy in such a way as to enhance the likelihood of achieving desired outcomes, and I recognize this as a strategic skill set. Communication skills correlate strongly with those relational skills that are integral to the Caritas Processes— they impact not only the crucial conversations but also set the stage for meaningful and caring moments with staff. Using the Caritas Processes as a framework for leadership practice has deepened my relational skills. Initially, I wondered if I would become "too soft" (what does it mean to be too soft, anyway?). Concerns dissipated as I recognized that through caritas, I developed a greater clarity of role and values. Resultantly, I have more confidence in my abilities to effectively engage and navigate the diverse issues of the day-to-day— from the simple to the most complex.

Watson speaks of "opening to that which might be, not conforming to what already is and which no longer serves self or society" (2008, p. 21). Such is the case with health reform and the restructuring of the American healthcare system. Nurses, the most prevalent of healthcare providers, are invited to step into a new space and create new options. There is the promise of an unfolding of possibilities extending beyond the medico-techno model of care that has become the national standard but clearly no longer works. Nurse-driven models of care will be advanced to create access to care for millions of newly insured. Population health management, protocols and clinical practice guidelines, chronic disease coaching and management, shared visits, and telehealth all provide context for "being-doing-becoming nursing with a new tune, a new rhythm" (Watson,

2008, p. xxi). Seeing beyond the point of care becomes requisite, as the concept of care across the continuum is reconceived yet again.

Now I ponder the characteristics of an ambulatory care model in an academic medical center and recognize it as (too) highly influenced by the acute care environment in which we reside, and not sufficiently reflective of the communities in which our patients live. Watson compels me to see beyond the point of care and what *is*, and to strive to manifest what could be. Healthcare solutions of the future will significantly depend upon nursing. What do we, as nurses, bring to healthcare that is different? Where or when does health begin? In merely asking the questions, the limitations of the medico-techno model that has felt so constraining begin to loosen. Much about health occurs outside of an exam room. Where are we in this discussion—perhaps more importantly we must each ask ourselves, "Where am *I* in this discussion?" Health equity has become a driving value. There is significant potential for the discipline to influence a political agenda that addresses social determinants of health, including poverty, substandard education, homelessness, and issues of public safety. Where is our voice? Embracing an open-systems model and an eco-caring cosmology allows for new appreciation of the interconnectedness of it all—to each other, to the world, to the environment, and to self and society. In such a model (elements of which can be traced back to Florence Nightingale), the nurse sheds the constraints of the exam room to give voice, shifting the old and the new toward a broader sphere of influence—and in this context, nursing "owns the source of our own power and possibilities" (Watson, 2008, p. 21). Nurses discover the power to say, "I commit. I will give voice. I will illuminate the voices of those in need."

As my own caritas consciousness expands, I continue to recognize the need for nursing leadership but feel naturally less inclined for it to be hierarchical. I seek to create a culture of leadership that has greater alignment with the values of Caring Science, where staff feels supported to care for patients, rather than *managed*. Recently, while working closely with an administrative colleague in the development of an organizational chart for an ambulatory service line, I encouraged a transition from a model that was top-heavy and reporting-structure-focused to one that was relationship driven. The newer model, one that places patients at the top, followed by the front line staff supporting the patient, and then management, was a clear acknowledgment of caritas values—the patient is the primary driver in this care delivery model. Placing the management team beneath the staff reflects a caritas-informed leader's responsibility to support staff through transpersonal relationships rather than the traditional management model.

Transpersonal caring relationships are guided by an evolving caritas consciousness (Watson, 2008). Implicit in this is concern and recognition of other as embodied spirit. Interactions that are spirit-centered set the stage for a connection that transcends ego and the need for professional control (Watson, 2008). Initially intended for application to the nurse-patient relationship, the foundational concepts of transpersonal caring (open and sensitive to another, remaining within another's frame of reference, giving attention to subtleties and behavioral cues) are transferrable and have application within the role of a nursing director. Supporting the work of the staff to deliver excellent care to patients and families drives my practice. I strive to be authentic, present, and trustworthy. In a busy healthcare environment, with multiple competing demands, I acknowledge that I struggle with staying present. I now hold it as a value and thus work harder to achieve it.

Through Touchstones, I have come to value the concept of a *pause* and when cognizant, use it to impact equanimity, clarity of purpose, tenor, and tone. Increasingly, I find I am cultivating curiosity—my own and that of others. I seek to assume less and wonder more. Therapeutic use of self has been an effective way to guide and develop staff. I have become more willing to go beyond ego, to become a little more vulnerable, and to expose my own shortcomings to increase the value of, or the receptivity to, the teaching moment. I hope to inspire and encourage in those teachable moments, thereby elevating each to a caring moment. I now see the nursing staff from a more holistic lens, understanding and developing an interest in staff both personally and professionally. While applying such concepts to leadership—especially that of spirit-centeredness—is admittedly unconventional, my approach to practice from a caring literacy framework—whether problem-solving a staffing issue, coaching, or engaging in crucial conversations—has proven more effective.

Professional development has long been considered a hallmark of the nursing profession, and significant attention is often given to those scientific and more technical aspects of the role. However, caring literacy uniquely requires intentionally attending to or cultivating one's own sense of humanity and establishing a healing presence (Watson, 2008). In this sense, an evolved caring consciousness becomes counterpoint to the medico-technical skills that are most frequently reinforced. Through caring literacy, Watson tells us that our heart intelligence, centeredness, and intentionality have capacity to expand. This evolution of an expanded form of consciousness is rooted in a process of self-growth and awareness (Watson, 2008). Thus, through Caring Science, the concept of professional development is broadened to reflect a lifelong commitment to a caritas-literacy-informed practice and reflects a continuous need to nurture one's heart-centeredness. In my personal journey towards a caritas-informed practice, I recognized that competing demands within the work environment were impacting my ability to establish authentic presence when engaging with staff. I was aware of the problem and found it distressing. I recognized the need to quiet my busy mind and enhance my connectedness—both to self and other. The creation of an intentional stream of caring consciousness proved to be the antidote to my sense of being "too busy" when consistently applied. Practicing centering exercises, meditating, and the setting of daily intentions has helped create strong connections to staff and self, and further supports a greater congruence between stated goals and actions, while intentionally favoring those that support a culture of caring.

Through the Caritas Coaching program and implementation of a reflective practice, which includes meditation, HeartMath, tai chi, and other modalities, a personal sense of self-awareness has started to emerge. This transformative process has aided the development of clarity of values and purpose, changed a management style to a caritas-informed leadership style, and further enhanced professional and personal relationships while broadening relational skills. Through emerging awareness, the silence was sufficient to finally hear those inner longings that had once been forgotten but now seek to be expressed. A deep appreciation for the value of the caring moment has been cultivated—for the significance of that moment in the nurse-patient experience, but also for the potential of caring moments to transform an organization. With Caring Science as the foundation, a truly patient-centered transformation of the healthcare system can be undertaken. This energizes me and restores my connection to the patient, the staff, and the organization. There is an inherent resilience that one encounters through caring. I begin again, dreaming of "possibilities not yet dreamt of—vibrating possibilities...for humanity, for health and for healing" (Watson, p. xix, 2008).

FINAL REFLECTIONS

The American healthcare system is experiencing challenging times, and today much about the future may feel uncertain. Human caring theory can serve as a compass, guiding us toward that which is timeless and should remain a constant—caring. Watson's interlude reminds nursing to "turn toward love and caring from one's own 'deep self'" (Watson, 2008, p. xix). With large numbers of patients seeking access to care and the infusion of technology into our care delivery models, we will indeed be propelled into creating new options for health and healing. However, the most important work we will ever do is not technical and cannot be prescribed, and waits to be discovered in those caring moments occurring in our hospitals and clinics—everyday miracles. Through cultivating those moments with intentionality, we are offered the opportunity to reconnect meaningfully to the eternal sacredness of our caring work for humanity. "Love is the highest level of consciousness and the greatest source of healing in the world" (Watson, 2008, p. 40). The world needs it. *Be* it.

REFERENCE

Watson, J. (2008). *Nursing: The philosophy and science of caring* (rev. ed.). Boulder, CO: University Press of Colorado.

CARING LEADERSHIP AS A CARITAS COACH

–Christine Buckley, DNP, MBA, BSN, RN, CPHQ, NEA-BC, Caritas Coach

Christine reveals in this chapter how Caring Science guides her in her formal leadership role as a nurse manager in creating a caring professional practice environment. Christine emphasizes the importance of attending to her own journey of continuous becoming as a foundation for nurturing an environment that fosters human connectedness for staff, patients, and families. She explores how Caring Science–the foundation for her leadership practice–provides a structure and language for relating to others, and provides vivid examples of caritas in action that illuminate what it means to embody Caring Science.

CHRISTINE'S CARITAS JOURNEY

For me, becoming a Caritas Coach has meant cultivating an awareness of my humanity and the interconnectedness of all aspects of life. Caring Science provides a structure and language to better grasp all aspects of caring theory and the caring-healing modalities that draw caring theory into our everyday activities. Through this framework, I can clearly identify caring qualities and foster an increased awareness of those qualities—for myself and for my staff.

As a Caritas Coach and in my current role of Associate Chief Nurse for maternal child health and specialty services, ongoing attention to the development of caritas literacies offers a beacon. The 10 Caritas Processes provide a comprehensive review of caritas goals and literacies—ways of being, becoming, doing, and knowing. These are important; without a clear destination, we are less likely to end up where we want to go.

Practicing as a Caritas Coach and caring leader is a day-to-day—often minute-to-minute—exercise. Although my intention is to be a caritas leader at all times, I often fall short. However, I have discovered that by clearly setting that intention and incorporating the language of caritas into my daily activities, I am more likely to succeed. The language and direction provided by the Caritas Processes not only inform how I embody caring qualities, but also provide a structure to continue to explore and support my personal efforts to integrate caring literacy into everyday actions. As someone in a leadership role, this approach helps me to recognize and nurture these ways of being in the workplace, setting the stage for caring literacy and creating a ripple of caritas throughout the team.

I have also set a conscious intention to support direct caregivers. The primary mission of most healthcare organizations is to provide compassionate and expert care to patients and families. However, we must also explicitly articulate care of the nursing staff as an equally important goal. In fact, care of staff is essential when fostering an environment that consistently meets the needs of patients and families.

Of course, without leaders who model caring behaviors, we can hardly expect our staff to exhibit them. As a Caritas Coach, it is my responsibility to model these behaviors. It is also my job to bring this critical caritas work forward to engage in nursing's deepest roots, connect with its essence in a way that supports caregivers, and build an environment that fosters human connectedness and better meets the needs of patients, families, and providers. With these aims in mind, I work to:

- Engage in transpersonal caring through intentional practice
- Clearly *see* staff
- Connect with self and other
- Engage in mindful and reflective practice

TRANSPERSONAL CARING THROUGH INTENTIONAL PRACTICE

Transpersonal caring is the cornerstone of Caring Science and the path to incorporating the concepts of Caring Science into our daily lives. Transpersonal caring relationships have been described as the foundation of Watson's work (Sitzman & Watson, 2013, p. 17). For me, cultivating an understanding of transpersonal caring has been crucial.

Dr. Watson often discusses the importance of intentionality in our work and in our lives, particularly from the perspective of our shared humanity (Watson, 1997; Watson, 1999; Watson, 2008). Intentionality is also a key aspect of transpersonal caring. If I am meeting with a staff member or colleague about an issue or problem, I set an intention for that meeting. For example, when meeting with a staff member to discuss performance areas in need of improvement, I set an intention to deliver the information sensitively and respectfully while honoring all of the person's contributions and good qualities. I try to put myself in the person's shoes, to be open to hearing what he or she may have to say, and to remember that this information may be difficult for the person to hear. I want to present the information in such a way that it is not perceived as criticism, but as an opportunity. This helps us act as partners, finding the best way to move forward together successfully.

Recently I presided over a debriefing after a difficult clinical event involving a child. Although the outcome of this event was ultimately positive, things did not go as planned. The event revealed clear opportunities for improvement as a team. As the group converged for the meeting, there was palpable tension in the air. Some of the staff involved in the event had been quite distraught by its unfolding and had been vocal in their views about how it had been managed by their colleagues.

Before the debriefing, I set an intention to honor the dedication and commitment of all team members. Knowing that all staff were concerned about the patient and family, I opened the meeting by acknowledging the shared intention of the team to provide the best possible care and by updating the group on the patient's improving condition. Then I highlighted the teamwork and skill exhibited by the entire team before noting the need to discuss our opportunities to improve. This seemed to settle the group. It also united us in our intention to make things better as we moved forward together. The ensuing discussion was respectful. It focused on the issues at hand, setting the stage for a satisfying resolution. We acknowledged our common intention and articulated what was in our hearts, allowing us to reclaim our shared purpose and demonstrate transpersonal caring.

CLEARLY SEEING

The first step toward intentionality is awareness. With a foundation of awareness in place, I am better able to observe transpersonal caring moments throughout the day and to acknowledge nurses and other staff who participate in these moments. I find that staff members are often grateful to be recognized in this way, and this recognition helps them to grasp the impact of these moments on their patients, their colleagues, and themselves. Seeing and acknowledging caring moments with staff and colleagues also helps others see these moments more clearly. The ultimate outcome, in Watson's words, is that "caring and love beget caring and love" (Watson, 2008, p. 87).

All healthcare providers—nurses included—play a vital role at the bedside, providing direct care for patients and families. Truly *seeing* all staff helps set the stage for a caring culture that supports caregivers so they are empowered to attend to the sacred work of patient care. It's an essential way to honor their experience, while reminding them of the critical impact they have on patient healing and the care environment.

One way that nurse leaders can convey that they clearly see their staff is by providing the time, space, and support to perform self-care—for example, coordinating coverage to give a staff member a much-needed break or providing food when staff might be hungry. So too are debriefs following difficult events. A debrief provides a dynamic forum to discuss an event from the perspective of the staff and an opportunity to access additional support services for an individual or the team.

Nurse leaders can also demonstrate that they see—and hear—their nurses by recognizing when they are under stress and responding with authentic caring. At times I have seen excellent nurses exhibit signs of overwhelming stress. This often manifests in uncaring attitudes or behaviors toward patients, families, colleagues, or self. Overwhelming stress may also result in poor communication or ineffective decision-making, affecting teamwork and the practice environment (Shirey, Ebright, & McDaniel, 2013; Shirey, 2007; Judkins, 2004). As a Caritas Coach and nurse leader, it's incumbent upon me to acknowledge the stress and frustration experienced by nurses while respectfully and collaboratively addressing the issues and behaviors that result. This allows nurses to feel seen and heard.

Connecting with Self and Others

Becoming a Caritas Coach has afforded me the opportunity to learn the meaning and language of caritas. This language helps us connect with our deepest selves and resonate with our core essence. This synergy of words and sentiment is as essential to our spirit as the alignment of our muscles and spinal column with our body. Just as misalignment in the body may lead to significant pain or mobility problems, using words that don't reflect our actions (or vice versa) can have a powerful negative effect. Through my Caritas Coach education, I have become much more aware of the power words have to transform my perspective. Incorporating meaningful and descriptive words into my day—such as *compassion, peace,* and *mindfulness*—serves as a reminder and grounding force in my Caring Science work. These words connect me with myself, in turn helping me to connect with others.

Early on I was shy about discussing topics around caring literacy and connecting with self and others. I have begun to lose my shyness around these topics, however. I have even learned to judiciously incorporate the "L word" (love). We readily admit to loving an article of clothing, a haircut, or a particular food. Why are we reluctant to acknowledge our love for each other?

The same goes for gratitude. I have found that gratitude is a powerful caring-healing practice both personally and professionally. People in every healthcare environment experience stressful times and difficult situations. However, maintaining a level of awareness and identifying when gratitude is an appropriate sentiment can have a unifying positive effect.

Since I have begun speaking about these topics, more people have acknowledged these issues and encouraged me to discuss them than I expected. It is as if we all need to be given permission to discuss these most basic experiences and shared vulnerabilities. Within the caritas community, I find the freedom to use these words—words like love—and express related feelings of joy more liberally.

MINDFUL AND REFLECTIVE PRACTICE

Throughout the course of each day, many challenges affect our sense of equanimity. It takes dedicated practice and sometimes substantial personal reserves to withstand the storm of events faced by nursing and healthcare leaders in the day-to-day healthcare environment.

As a caring leader and Caritas Coach, I must attend to my own journey—my *continuous becoming*—to meet these challenges. Significant ongoing attention to my own self-care is a vital component of this work. Without conscious attention to self-care, awareness becomes blurry or may be lost entirely. Practicing self-care also serves as a model for others.

Self-care must be the first step in any plan to guide and sustain a Caring Science practice; it is essential for any nurse or nurse leader. A self-care program provides the foundation for caring literacy and a sense of equanimity—hallmarks of a Caritas Coach and a true leader. As Jean Watson writes, "truly the caring-healing dimensions of nursing are needed now more than ever" (Watson, 1999, p. xxi). Caritas serves not only as an invitation to care for self, but presents this as an imperative.

Practicing self-care means being kind to oneself. I believe kindness is a necessary (though at times overlooked) aspect of our busy lives. Practicing kindness toward ourselves improves our ability to be kind to others.

Self-care brings self-compassion and self-awareness. Just as the food we eat nourishes and supports our bodies, self-compassion and self-awareness feed our inner being. Self-compassion includes realizing our own vulnerabilities, frailties, and imperfections. Interestingly, this helps us to realize our interconnectedness. Self-awareness is critical to being fully and authentically present in any given moment—a key characteristic of a caring leader. Authentic presence is required for any nurse leader who seeks to compassionately and effectively operate in today's complex healthcare environment. Only by being authentically present can we truly engage with others.

Reflective practice is necessary to keep caring at the forefront of our thoughts and actions. Caring is not a one-time event or accomplishment. It is a work in progress and in constant need of attention. Vigilance is required to stay on course or to get back on track if the way is lost. I practice mindfulness—for example, focusing on my breath throughout the day and especially before, after, or even during a difficult encounter—to find my way back to caring.

FINAL REFLECTIONS

Writing about becoming a Caritas Coach has brought to mind an experience I had early in my caritas journey. It was while overseeing a self-care education and mindfulness pilot for nurses in our special care nursery. I had chosen this clinical area for the pilot because I had seen evidence of stress due to the challenging clinical and emotional demands of caring not only for babies born with narcotic abstinence syndrome but also their families, who were struggling in their own ways with the devastating effects of substance use disorder.

During the pilot, I met with night staff to review Watson's theory as the framework for the intervention. One nurse who had been on the unit for many years remarked, "That sounds like a lot of hooey." We laughed. I acknowledged that at times, the language can be a bit...convoluted. But then I talked about what concepts within the theory resonated with me.

Afterward, I asked for her thoughts. The nurse paused only briefly before agreeing that Watson's theory made sense and could apply in the clinical environment. This nurse went on to share with me that her son had committed suicide a year earlier and that she continued to struggle with her grief. Therefore, she was particularly interested in the focus on self-care and mindfulness. Moreover, she believed that her son—who had been a gifted mental-health counselor and had experienced significant stress in that role—might have benefited from education around these practices. Interactions like this one remind me of our interconnectedness and inspire me to continue to work to bring forth Caring Science.

> *"A moment of self-compassion can change your entire day. A string of such moments can change the course of your life."*
>
> –Christopher K. Germer

References

Judkins, S. K. (2004). Stress among nurse managers: Can anything help? *Nurse Researcher, 12*(2), 58–70.

Shirey, M. R. (2007). An evidence-based solution for minimizing stress and anger in nursing students. *Journal of Nursing Education, 46*(12), 568–571.

Shirey, M. R., Ebright, P. R., & McDaniel, A. M. (2013). Nurse manager cognitive decision-making amidst stress and work complexity. *Journal of Nursing Management, 21*(1), 17–30.

Sitzman, K., & Watson, J. (2013). *Caring science, mindful practice: Implementing Watson's human caring theory.* New York, NY: Springer Publishing Co.

Watson, J. (1997). The theory of human caring: Retrospective and prospective. *Nursing Science Quarterly, 10*(1), 49–52.

Watson, J. (1999). *Postmodern nursing and beyond.* London, UK: Churchill Livingstone.

Watson, J. (2008). *Nursing: The philosophy and science of caring* (rev. ed.). Boulder, CO: University Press of Colorado.

Creating and Sustaining a Caritas Way of Being

–Lacey Lefere, MSN, BA, RN, AHN-BC, C-EFM, Caritas Coach

Lacey describes her time in the Caritas Coach Education Program (CCEP) as a journey of self-discovery and renewal, helping her to practice with more confidence, consciousness, self-awareness, and authenticity. In this chapter, Lacey shares how Caring Science enables her to be intentional in her thoughts and actions, her relationships, and her perspectives on life. She uses this newfound way of being to coach others to realize their own potential with love and care.

Lacey's Caritas Journey

If asked why they opted to enter nursing, it is safe to say that most nurses would respond with some version of "to care for patients"—myself included. If we go on to ask nurses what it means to care, however, answers will likely be far more varied.

The meaning of caring is different for almost everyone. I've heard caring described in a variety of ways—the act of listening to someone, staying after one's regularly scheduled shift to finish a task, or sharing a story to better relate to a patient. Some say caring means taking all the necessary steps to keep someone alive. Others say caring means being present for someone as they are dying. I have also had people stop, think, and admit that they aren't sure *what* caring is.

It is in our attempt to define, quantify, qualify, explain, and advance caring that Caring Science and Watson's 10 Caritas Processes (Watson, 2008) come alive. Caring Science, and everything that accompanies it, serves as a language, practice model, definition, and standard for caring not only in healthcare but also in our world.

It is my experience that Caring Science finds some people, while others must seek it out. In my case, Caring Science found me. I was lucky to make my way to a Watson-affiliated hospital early in my career. Becoming a Caritas Coach was also something that found me. It was not something to which I aspired. Indeed, I didn't even know what it was until I was asked to participate in the CCEP. Prior to completing the CCEP, I told people it was a program that would help me become more conscious of Watson's Caring Science philosophy in my work. Although that answer was not incorrect, I now tell people that my participation in the CCEP has ensured that I will remain in nursing for many years to come.

One beautiful thing about being a Caritas Coach is that each of us sets our own "job description." That is, we all define how the principles of Caring Science will apply in our life at work, at home, and beyond. My current roles as clinical nurse specialist, wife, friend, daughter, and Christian (to name a few) both complement and are enhanced by the concepts of Caring Science and, more specifically, my role as a Caritas Coach. I participate in a wonderful and diverse caritas community filled with like-minded people whose goals are as similar to mine as they are unique. In other words, we are all working toward the same aim, but we will get there in our own ways.

A MORE CONSCIOUS WAY OF BEING

Becoming a Caritas Coach taught me a lot about Caring Science, the 10 Caritas Processes, authentic presence, healing environments, and transpersonal caring moments (Watson, 2008). As much as I learned about all these concepts, though, what I learned about myself was just as important. Becoming a Caritas Coach challenged me to expand my way of thinking and develop a more conscious way of being.

I believe there are many paths to self-discovery and renewal, and that the path each of us takes depends on any number of variables. My path to becoming a Caritas Coach easily aligned with how I approached life in terms of my religion and spirituality, wellness, literacy, and occupation. I was able to learn and incorporate caritas literacy at my own individualized learning curve and pace. Being a "shining light" or a "lit candle in a dark room" were common analogies used during my upbringing. As I have grown older, it has been difficult at times to remain strong enough to shine my light on what I deem to be true in the face of adversity. Becoming a Caritas Coach gave me the tools to generate that spark of caring light to shine in my life at home, at work, and in my community.

A Caritas Coach embodies and lives the values of Caring Science in a way that shines a light on self, others, the community, and the world. This might seem like a heavy burden. But even as being a Caritas Coach places this burden on us, it lifts the burden by emphasizing self-care. A Caritas Coach is comfortable caring for self through practices like self-reflection and personal exploration.

Indeed, it is through these exercises that the Caritas Coach with the greatest potential for human caring is born.

For me, the shift to Caring Science practice and thought patterns lies in recognizing that my ultimate goal is to move to a caritas or Caring Science way of being. When this happens, I will no longer need to consciously infuse my practice and thinking with Caring Science. Rather, it will happen automatically. It will become less about what I *do* in my practice and everyday life and more about my presence in each moment. This will occur through the constant and continual work I put into my own self-care and self-awareness. Through this work on self, we create our own unique worldview that enables and guides our thinking, practice, development, and sustainment of care. Caring Science gives me unlimited permission to focus on caring for self to better care for those around me.

CARITAS CONNECTEDNESS

While I'm at work, my goal as a Caritas Coach is to bring a quantifiable, tangible language of caring to almost everything I do. I use the lens and language of Caring Science to shape policies, research, associate education, patient care plans, unit and project goals, and more. I infuse the 10 Caritas Processes into my communications with associates, into hiring interviews, and into new-employee orientation procedures. Each day, my attention to Caring Science influences my patience with, compassion for, prioritization and evaluation of, and presence to every item on my to-do list. This influence only grows stronger as I tend to my own self-care and balance. Therefore, the degree to which Caring Science affects my thinking and practice always depends on me. Fortunately, as a Caritas Coach, I am now able to call on my own heart energy more effectively when things become stressful at work.

Caring Science also affects my relationships at home and in my community. I did not expect this when I agreed to become a Caritas

Coach. Although I understood at a basic level that each aspect of my life—my work life, home life, church life, and so on—touched the others, I had effectively compartmentalized them. I lacked the caritas consciousness that instills awareness of the impact and influence of each piece of my life on the others. Now I more fully grasp how my state of being at work can influence the interactions I have with my husband at home, the energy I bring when meeting up with friends, even the food I cook for dinner or my ability to sleep—the list goes on. Caring Science has helped me merge the separate areas of my life and more effectively transition from one thing to another.

I also recognize that each day brings opportunities in my work and home life to be more considerate of Caring Science and the 10 Caritas Processes. Conversations (verbal and non-verbal), emails, processes, policies, prioritization, conflict resolution, and many other encounters and events offer me openings as a nursing leader, wife, and member of society to integrate and interact in caring-conscious ways.

Caring Science reminds us that we cannot live our lives in a series of silos—work, home, community, world, and so on. But we also see this elsewhere. Some religions, different studies of human interaction, and even social media outlets remind us that we are all linked. Understanding the connection, integration, and interdependence of these silos is key to understanding the theory of Caring Science. In our high-tech world, it is becoming easier to see the connectedness of the world we live in. But—ironic as it may seem—it is becoming harder and harder to see the interdependent nature of our world. Many people recognize that if they post something on Facebook, a thousand people may see it. But they fail to recognize that a thousand people may also feel the residual impact of that action. Caring Science calls us to intentionally acknowledge, today and tomorrow, the impact that all thoughts, words, and actions have on our world and universe.

SEEING THE OPPORTUNITIES IN VULNERABILITY

For me, the most notable examples of the embodiment of Caring Science involve vulnerability. This is because Caring Science interprets vulnerability not as weakness or helplessness but as a positive opportunity for transition.

This became clear to me during an incident at work. Shortly after assuming an interim management role, I recognized that there was significant conflict between two members of the team, with misalignment regarding role expectations. This resulted in tension that created an uneasy work environment for everyone in the department. To resolve this situation, I called for a mediation session. I hadn't expected to hold a mediation session so early in my transition to this role, and I did not feel very confident about doing it. I knew it would likely be difficult for those involved—and that it would be new and uncomfortable for me, too. Still, I assembled the two individuals along with a dependable third party who was better attuned than I to the day-to-day operations of this department.

Before becoming a Caritas Coach, I would have done three things differently. First, I would have thought that asking for support from a third party would be a sign of weakness. In fact, it was an opportunity to develop trust and use the knowledge of others. Second, I would have failed to create an intentional space for the private expression of thoughts and feelings. And third, I would have become very frustrated during the mediation and therefore unable to guide the conversation in a caring, healing way. As it was, though, I was able to help both individuals find clarity about their respective roles and determine how to move forward—and to do so in such a way that neither of them felt hurt or victimized. As a result, the work environment was vastly improved for all in the department. And I—by staying centered, grounded, and self-aware throughout the experience—was able to leave the interaction without feeling completely depleted of my own internal resources.

TRANSPERSONAL CARING

Before my journey to becoming a Caritas Coach, my attempt to define transpersonal caring would have started with me searching the Internet for the phrase "transpersonal caring" and ended with me saying that I care very much and try to make it show in everything I do. While the second part of this statement still holds true, Caring Science has given me a language to better communicate how caring translates into my practice. I see transpersonal caring as something that stems from being open to the unknown possibility and potential of our interactions with others as we operate through the lens of Caring Science.

Because I no longer work in a direct-care bedside nursing position, I focus on manifesting transpersonal caring while supporting those who *are* at the bedside. I take the energy I used to pour into my patients' hospital experiences and pour it into my peers' work experiences. I strive to align my work with theirs to help them create transpersonal caring moments with our patients. I strive to help others to realize their impact and potential in the field of nursing, and to guide them toward maximizing those gifts and talents.

Transpersonal caring moments emerge between my team and me in many forms. They occur most often when an associate comes to me to voice a concern, suggest a change, or seek advice. When an associate expresses a concern, I give the person a safe space to share his or her feelings while sustaining a loving-trusting relationship. When one suggests a change, I guide a genuine teaching-learning experience by acknowledging the artistry of the caring-healing process from all perspectives. And when one asks for advice, I take care to listen intentionally with loving-kindness and to foster an environment that allows for the other's own emergence and development. Through each of these, I practice authentic presence. That is, I give my full and undivided attention. By grounding and centering, I also ensure that any emotion in the exchange does not cloud my end of the interaction. I use the 10 Caritas Processes to create a nonjudgmental and agenda-free environment to allow for the expansion of consciousness for all involved and a transpersonal caring-healing interaction.

I also work to bring transpersonal caring to meetings and interactions I have with those who are no longer at the bedside, and to those with whom I do not work on a regular basis. I can think of many times when associates I do not work with and do not know personally have opened up to me in beautiful and unexpected ways. I believe these experiences are the result of simple actions like walking down the hall with a smile, making eye contact and saying hello, and being open to the unknown opportunity—even miracle—that each passing interaction holds.

My ability to navigate the field of healthcare, sustain my caring practices, and advance in perceived power and rank mean nothing if I do not create a positive ripple through my interactions and choices. I am where I am today because someone saw something in me even before I did. The caritas journey is a good example of something for which "you get out what you put in," but for me it started with someone else taking that first step. My work as a Caritas Coach calls me to take similar first steps for others.

COMBATING BURNOUT WITH CARITAS LITERACY

Earlier I said that participating in the CCEP is what will keep me in nursing for years to come. To elaborate, I believe that if I had not developed caring literacy, I would have grown frustrated by my lack of a language to describe my feelings, goals, ideas, and aspirations as they relate to nursing and my role in it. Not only that, I believe I would have lacked the tools needed to support myself through the changes and challenges that accompany promotion and advancement. Frustration, exhaustion, stress, and burnout might very well have gotten the best of me.

The greatest tools I've added to my toolbox during my caritas journey are patience, an ability to ground and center myself, permission to practice self-care, and an expanded consciousness. These effectively enable me to be a positive beacon of light in every aspect (or silo) of my world. The journey was not—*is* not—always easy. Some view the act of grounding and centering, which occurs through practices like intentional breathing, as a weakness. But I know these practices allow for greater effectiveness and resilience, so I've disciplined myself to continue them. To make time for self-care, I have had to make sacrifices. And an expanded consciousness can be extremely overwhelming without appropriate self-care and a mentor to help guide the process.

I used to justify avoidance behaviors by saying it was easier to not get involved. Caritas literacy has changed that. With caritas literacy I have gotten better at welcoming the unknown and embracing the discomfort that comes with something new. I can more intentionally and insightfully use the feelings and emotions elicited by different experiences to help guide me from point A to point B.

TRUSTING THE PROCESS

Some people have rigid timelines for their careers, conferences, classes, promotions, locations, etc. I used to be one of those people. Although this approach is not necessarily wrong, I have learned through caring literacy that it is not the best approach for me. As I take steps in my own professional development, caring literacy enables me to "trust the process."

When asked about my career goals and plans, I can now say with confidence that I work every day to put myself in positions in which I am challenged to learn something new while supporting the greater good. When I find myself at a crossroads, I can now use caring language and concepts to analyze the pros and cons of each possible choice.

I believe that by taking this approach, I will be best equipped for whatever opportunity comes my way in the future. I believe I will be presented with opportunities that fit my skills and personality. I also believe this approach allows for the greatest potential for true happiness and fulfillment. I still set goals, but rather than feeling completely derailed when things do not go according to plan, I see opportunities in the new situation.

REFLECTING WITH INTENTION

Self-awareness and reflection are two of the most critical practices in Caring Science. In my case, self-awareness and reflection enable me to maintain a relatively stable personal baseline. That is, these tools give me the ability to ride the highs and lows of the day-to-day without letting them consume me. It is from this baseline that growth and progress are possible.

Throughout my life I have always readily used reflection as a tool for growth. I have learned through my caritas journey, however, that simply thinking about things is not enough. Taking the next step to more intentional reflective practices, such as journaling, is key. Although this has not come easily to me, I am committed to the practice, as I have found it to be a critical component of caring. Intentional reflection has helped me organize and process the increased information load that comes with an expanded consciousness and increased self-awareness.

Increased self-awareness has been integral to not only identifying the need for reflection in my day-to-day practice but also giving myself the permission to do so. Through exercises in reflection, I have improved my self-awareness. These two practices are synergistic. They work together to act as the glue that binds the art and science of nursing practice. As a result, the art of what I do as a nurse emerges and works with—rather than against—the science of our traditional medical model.

Reflection has helped me reveal my hopes and dreams as a person and a professional. Self-awareness has allowed me the openness and vulnerability to acknowledge and work toward these hopes and dreams. I use the phrase "hopes and dreams" intentionally. It calls to mind the mystery of being truly open to the universal possibility of Caring Science. This state of *being* rather than *doing* is the light that I, as a Caritas Coach, hope to shine in every aspect of my life, forever and beyond.

FINAL REFLECTIONS

Throughout my life I have participated in many personal and professional development exercises. All these left me feeling great—but only for a short time. The same happened when I first encountered Caring Science. For me, Caring Science was a useful answer to theoretical nursing questions but not so much a universal way of being. I struggled to get deep enough into Caring Science to cultivate a truly sustainable worldview of caring. When I became a Caritas Coach, my awareness and consciousness began to expand. I was suddenly able to apply Caring Science in personally meaningful and renewing ways.

My journey through Caring Science and becoming a Caritas Coach has been one of great self-discovery and acceptance. Having a better understanding of who I am and where I stand within the framework of caring concepts has enabled me to better shine light and offer hope in situations I might previously have avoided. I have reset my default to more inclusively examine and consider all perspectives of a situation—not just at work, but at home and in my community as well. Finally, I can better maintain coherence and resilience with less conscious effort, thereby generating a much higher level of personal and professional satisfaction.

REFERENCE

Watson, J. (2008). *Nursing: The philosophy and science of caring* (rev. ed.). Boulder, CO: University Press of Colorado.

Working with Others Within the Context of Caring Relationships

–Nancy Mathews, MS, BS, Caritas Coach, HeartMath Trainer

With an expertise in continuing education, Nancy explores in this chapter how she came to embrace Caring Science for personal and professional growth. A caregiver from outside the nursing profession, Nancy shares how this theory helped her to develop self-awareness, practice self-care, and cultivate open and authentic communication. Although her journey is relatively new, she clearly articulates the value of caring literacy and its potential for healing self and nurturing transpersonal relationships with others.

NANCY'S CARITAS JOURNEY

"Authentic caring relationship building is concerned with deepening our humanity; it is about processes of being-becoming more humane, compassionate, aware, and awake to our own and other's human dilemma." (Watson, 2008, p. 72)

From an early age, I had a caring, compassionate, and loving nature. I was born in Sycamore, Illinois, the youngest of four children. When I was 9, a career opportunity for my father brought my family to South America. We moved first to Valencia, Venezuela. Later, we moved to Sao Paulo, Brazil, where I graduated from high school. Afterward, I returned to the United States to go to college. In 1980 I graduated from the University of Wisconsin-Milwaukee with an undergraduate degree in sociology. I then earned a master's degree in computer information systems.

While in South America, I experienced different cultures. I learned to respect diversity and the value of being kind. I also developed a strong work ethic. This work ethic led me to pursue leadership positions in business and academia to complement a personal life full of adventures. As life became more complex and challenging, however, I realized something wasn't right. At home, I cared for others at the expense of caring for myself. At work, I struggled to navigate professional bureaucracies and began to change jobs more frequently. As the years went by I remained unfilled and uncertain as to why. It wasn't until a few years ago, after a life-changing personal loss, that I was awakened to an opportunity to transform not only what I was doing, but my way of being.

My journey paralleled Jon Kabat-Zinn's famous book, *Wherever You Go, There You Are: Mindfulness Meditation in Everyday Life* (2005). This book emphasizes the importance of looking within and using our inner guiding light to navigate our journey rather than searching elsewhere for answers. Peace and satisfaction are something we carry with us, not something we obtain from other people or external circumstances. For many years, I relied on happiness and personal satisfaction from external sources instead of discovering my inner self and happiness from within.

In 2015 I began working for the Watson Caring Science Center at the University of Colorado. Drawn to the ethics and values of Caring Science, I wanted to use my knowledge and expertise in continuing education, technology, and course development to further the work of Caring Science in the world. I quickly realized that to deepen my ability to work in this area, I needed to become a Caritas Coach. I enrolled in the Caritas Coach Education Program (CCEP). I began to explore myself from within and to seek answers about the purpose and meaning of my life.

While immersing myself in Caring Science, I was also reading about mindfulness and exploring meditation. I was struck by the following quote:

> To allow ourselves to be truly in touch with where we already are, no matter where that is, we have got to pause in our experience long enough to let the moment sink in; long enough to actually feel the present moment, to see it in its fullness, to hold it in awareness and thereby come to know and understand it better. Only then can we accept the truth of this moment of our life, learn from it, and move on. (Kabat-Zinn, 2005, pp. xiii–xiv)

Mindfulness meditation has been an influential factor in my transformation; so too has fully embracing and practicing the 10 Caritas Processes. These offer language and guidance for deepening the inner self and radiating an open-hearted love and compassion for self and others.

It was not until I became a Caritas Coach that I understood how Caring Science deepens my ability to care and provides literacy to influence my actions within myself and with others. As I deepen my caring intentions, embrace altruistic values, and practice loving-kindness for myself and others, my inner purpose and commitment to human caring have become clearer and my way of being has begun to transform.

At the same time, I have developed interests in holistic approaches such as yoga, meditation, and Reiki. Learning new skills requires practice. It also opens my heart, sparks my creativity and growth, and encourages me to continue my Caring Science journey. These practices also help me connect with my source and assimilate my caring values with meaning and purpose in life.

I now realize that the gifts and answers lie within. I also recognize that the greatest challenges lead to the most rewarding accomplishments. The caritas values and processes continue to guide and sustain me through difficult times while helping me transform in a multitude of positive ways both personally and professionally. Most importantly, self-awareness, self-care practices, and authentic communication have helped me grow as a Caritas Coach and as a person.

PRACTICING SELF-CARE AND AWARENESS

> As a beginning, we have to learn how to offer
> caring, love, forgiveness, compassion and mercy
> to ourselves before we can offer authentic caring
> and love to others...explore how our unique gifts,
> talents, and skills can be translated into compassion-
> ate human caring-healing service for self and others.
> (Watson, 2008, p. 41)

Caring for myself has been one of my greatest challenges. But it is an important first step toward thoughtful and empathetic communication and relationships. This became clear to me when circumstances forced me to spend considerable time navigating the healthcare system to find proper care for my parents. In caring for them, I allowed little time to care for myself. Not surprisingly, my mind and body broke down from fatigue. Without caring literacy and caring-healing practices to sustain me, I became exhausted.

Talking with others in the CCEP, I quickly realized I wasn't the only one who sidestepped self-care. Self-care was a foreign concept to many of us. Yet I grasped that it was key to the caritas journey. Finally seeing myself as someone who cared for others at the expense of caring for myself was illuminating. I realized that to embrace Caring Science, I would have to learn to care for myself. Engaging in caring literacy through reading, reflecting, authentically conversing with others, and initiating intentional self-care practices facilitated my journey. It provided a balance between giving and receiving and the equanimity to manage challenging situations.

During chaotic and challenging times, my mind often becomes stormy with negative thoughts. I become unable to open space to cultivate the beautiful treasures of the present moment—awareness, compassion, life's miracles, and caring relationships. Mindful self-care practices such as meditation, yoga, and Reiki help center me and provide a balance between my inner feelings and emotions and life challenges. In particular, Reiki—a spiritual energy and holistic healing system for restoring physical and emotional well-being—has increased my spiritual awareness; I am currently in training to become a Reiki practitioner. I also practice self-care before settling in for the evening. I read, journal, meditate, or watch inspiring videos. Being centered and present in the moment helps me reflect more clearly and enhances my creativity. This in turn helps me consciously radiate loving-kindness to myself and others. Through these practices I find inner peace. Developing harmony within directly influences my self-awareness, allows for a restful sleep, and supports me in setting my intentions to meaningfully connect with others each day.

BEING PRESENT, AUTHENTIC, AND OPEN

Kornfield reinforces the need to understand our individual and collective contributions to a healthy culture within the context of Caring Science (1993, 2009). In other words, we might have all the wisdom and knowledge in the world, but if we can't embody this knowledge and wisdom through compassion, love, and kindness, we cannot be fully present or develop a spiritual connection with others. Similarly, Watson writes "without attending and cultivating one's own spiritual growth, insight, mindfulness, and spiritual dimension of life, it is very difficult to be sensitive to self and other. Without this lifelong process and journey, we can become hardened and brittle and can close down our compassion and caring for self and other" (Watson, 2008, p. 67).

Writing about being fully present reminds me of a growth opportunity I experienced with a colleague. After several months of working with her, I sensed a slight change in our communication. It would have been easy to ignore the change, assuming time would resolve it. But the CCEP taught me to open space for compassionate dialogue—so I did. During our conversation I discovered my colleague's concern: "Sometimes when you are with me, I feel you are half-listening—focusing on other things." Given my tendency to multitask, this did not surprise me. I often talk on the phone while checking my email, listen to conversations while focusing on other thoughts, and so on. These behaviors rob me of the opportunity to develop quality relationships and deepen my humanity. I realized that simply being present is not necessarily *being present*—with awareness and compassion. I vowed to do better.

In addition to working toward being present, I remain mindful of how I express myself—my tone of voice, choice of words, and nonverbal gestures. All these aspects affect how my message is received. This has helped me communicate more clearly and honestly. Before engaging in conversations with others, I take a few minutes to practice self-awareness—breathing, centering, and opening my

mind and heart. During the conversation, rephrasing words and gestures, monitoring my tone, and using caring body language help me
build relationships based in loving-kindness, compassion, trust, and
authenticity. Instead of trying to control the conversation, I work to
be authentically present; to listen; to use thoughtful, compassionate,
and nondefensive language; to hear the other's perspective; to ask
questions; and to encourage feedback. If the conversation drifts in
the wrong direction, I suggest we pause, take a minute to be silent
and reflect, allowing us to witness the dignity and humanity of the
other. By setting an intention to collaborate and share experiences
with others and allowing for the expression of both positive and
negative feelings, we create new space for compassion, knowledge,
diversity, awareness, and learning.

Even the medium used affects communication. Contemporary
work environments rely on technology (such as telephone, email,
and social media) rather than face-to-face dialogue for communication. This creates many interpersonal challenges. For example, a
recent email from a colleague announced a change in policy that I
found misguided. In the past I would have assertively questioned this
change. Instead, I responded using my caritas skills. First, instead
of challenging the policy in an email, I recommended we schedule
a time to meet in person. Then, during our face-to-face dialogue, I
strove to embody listening and compassion. In the end I came to better understand the other person's perspective. Exemplifying caring
behaviors, authentically listening, and asking questions provided an
open space for a shared knowledge exchange.

Reflecting on my life experiences from a Caring Science framework, I see the importance of open and authentic dialogue. This is
the foundation for trusting relationships. Refusing to allow experiences to change our behaviors, or changing our behaviors to avoid
conflict, leaves us in the shallow shoals of self. For years I avoided
difficult conversations to preserve harmony. I withheld my feelings
and emotions to avoid hurting others or to gain acceptance. This
was my norm for dealing with conflicts of any kind. One of my life
challenges has been overcoming this tendency to withhold. After

studying Caring Science, reading self-awareness books, and engaging in daily mindful practices, I realized that by withholding my authentic feelings, I deprive myself of learning and of an opportunity to make a difference in the world. Since then there have been several occasions on which I have allowed myself to be vulnerable and shared my experiences with others. Months after these interactions, many of these individuals told me that my insight and honesty made a difference in their lives. I am grateful for these moments. They help me grow.

As an aside, I use journaling as a means of self-discovery and to gather the courage to communicate more openly. Through journaling I explore my thoughts, reflections, and feelings; discover hidden lessons; and develop the courage to outwardly be the individual who lives within. Journaling my experiences has not only provided self-awareness, but also given me the audacity to engage in difficult authentic conversations—the key to trusting relationships.

I must also work to ensure others feel free to be their full selves with me—and that I take the time to truly *see* them. Recently, I attended a memorial service for a colleague who had been very reserved and quiet. I admit I didn't really know this man. During the service, the man's family and friends described him as someone who possessed great love and compassion—qualities many of us who worked with him never took the time to explore. "What a beautiful person," we said afterward. "I wish I had taken the time to know him."

Ultimately, Caring Science has increased my awareness of the importance of reaching outside my comfort zone, finding the beauty that is all around me, and opening my heart to learn from these wonderful hidden treasures.

Moving Forward on the Caring Journey

As I continue to embody Caring Science, facing my inner feelings and emotions while also confronting my life challenges, I more intentionally push myself to reflect on questions such as the following:

- Do I embody self-care practices, opening space to allow new ways of being and doing?

- Am I listening and being authentically present, truly engaging in dialogue, accepting with an open heart and open mind the true essence of the message within?

- Do I judge others before opening new space for listening, reflecting, learning, understanding, and growing?

- Where are my opportunities to manifest love, compassion, equanimity, and openness?

- Before engaging in a conversation, do I pause, open my heart, and engage my beginner's mind for new opportunity and growth, focusing my intention on humanity and dignity for all instead of personal outcomes or gains?

- Do I converse in a way that honors the diversity of another's opinions, allowing that person to be heard without judgment and taking time to understand the person's view, before providing mindful feedback that is caring and non-defensive?

- Do I model Caring Science as a leader even in structured and controlled organizational cultures?

- Do I balance love, compassion, and equanimity while challenging uncaring acts and behaviors?

Reflecting on my inner strengths and growth, I now realize as a Caritas Coach the importance of advancing these caring attributes one step further—to be all-encompassing "life-giving, life-receiving, human-to-human, spirit-to-spirit connection" (Watson, 2008, p. 73). Building trusting relationships based on authentic presence and love for myself and others is the foundation for being a Caritas Coach.

FINAL REFLECTIONS

Having heart-centered experiences with colleagues, nurturing my personal growth through Caring Science literacy, engaging in daily self-care, and having open and authentic communication have been instrumental in my development and growth. As I continue to apply the philosophy, values, and ethics of Caring Science in my life, I realize the intrinsic value of this theory and its transformational effects on the world. Spreading caring and love to others is like planting a seed that grows and reproduces, scattering beauty throughout the world.

Balancing Caring Science with daily life is often hard. Yet acknowledging and connecting with our deepest insecurities and vulnerabilities brings forth our humanity and supports Caring Science practices. For me, these practices have become the essence of my daily awareness and growth. They help me communicate in caring and authentic ways, open space for others to understand my intentions and wholeness within, and balance my inner and outer awareness. Although feelings and emotions still dominate my caring consciousness, my expanded inner awareness harnesses them to guide me toward harmony, compassion, love, and equanimity.

As a Caritas Coach, I see the importance of elevating what I have learned one step further by "being reflective, and mindful mid-step, mid-sentence, mid-action, when connecting with another person" (Watson, 2008, p. 73). By becoming a Caritas Coach and attempting to live the values and ethics of Caring Science every day, I have learned to appreciate the sacredness of my own personal and professional life. By doing so, I strive to be one of those seeds that flower, showering my own beauty, and empowering and nurturing others to do the same.

References

Kabat-Zinn, J. (2005). *Wherever you go, there you are: Mindfulness meditation in everyday life.* New York, NY: Hachette Book Group.

Kornfield, J. (1993). *A path with heart: A guide through the perils and promises of spiritual life.* New York, NY: Bantam.

Kornfield, J. (2009). *The wise heart: A guide to the universal teachings of Buddhist psychology.* New York, NY: Bantam.

Watson, J. (2008). *Nursing: The philosophy and science of caring* (rev. ed.). Boulder, CO: University Press of Colorado.

A Physician's Journey with Caritas: A Path to Healing

-Jennifer Reese, MD, Caritas Coach

Jenny was struck by the word *caritas* the first time she heard it, immediately recognizing it as the foundation not just of nursing but all of healthcare. Reflecting on the process of becoming a Caritas Coach, Jenny shares her deep dive into her own emotional and spiritual approaches to work and life. Jenny's story is not only about becoming a caritas doctor; it's about creating environments that support the resilience and well-being of all healthcare professionals.

JENNY'S CARITAS JOURNEY

The first time I heard the word *caritas,* I was sitting in a spirituality council meeting at our hospital. It resonated with me and I immediately wanted to learn more. A nurse colleague who was a Caritas Coach offered me a more detailed description of caritas. "This can't just be for nurses," I thought. "This is for everyone who works in healthcare."

As this discussion continued, we delved into practices of caritas, the science of caring, and ultimately the meaning of our work. We explored our calling as healthcare providers and the importance of being present during each experience with patients, their families, and our colleagues. During this same period, I was exploring my own spirituality, practicing authenticity and presence, and understanding self-care. It was a natural progression to implement this philosophy in my work as a pediatrician at a large academic medical center.

All around me I witnessed colleagues struggling with compassion fatigue, stress, and the impact of their constant exposure to suffering. I was struggling, too. I wanted to learn how to cope with this struggle and how we could become healthier as individuals and as teams to better care for our patients. This compelled me to become a Caritas Coach and in doing so to connect with my purpose, authenticity, values, and compassion.

Becoming a Caritas Coach takes commitment—of time and energy, and of self-awareness and openness to learning. For me, it also took a commitment to explore a new culture that is mostly composed of nurses. Although we work side by side and rely on each other, nurses and physicians speak different languages and have vastly different expectations and experiences. Therefore, integrating into this culture was also part of my caritas journey. I had the great fortune to participate in this process with nursing colleagues who embody passion, intelligence, patience, compassion, and most importantly a sense of humor.

The process of becoming a Caritas Coach involved a lot of reading and writing homework—something I hadn't had to do for years. But it also involved a refreshing deep dive into my emotional and spiritual approach to work and life. In particular, attending my first International Caritas Consortium opened my eyes to an expression of true compassion that I had never experienced in my work. Medical training is focused on acquiring knowledge and providing the right answers. It's about competition and achievement. Rarely do humility and compassion get overtly taught, or even recognized as admirable attributes.

Reading and learning a new language and approach to practice enabled me to identify what has now become my true calling: healing the healer. This is based on Caritas Process 1: "Practicing loving-kindness and equanimity for self and other" (Watson, 2008, p. 47). Perhaps this Caritas Process spoke to me because I had recently gone through a divorce and was struggling to balance my role as the mother of young children with my career and personal growth. I was facing head-on an opportunity to practice self-care, self-compassion, and healing. I was also inspired to help my colleagues alleviate their own suffering, whether due to personal or professional stressors. This laid the groundwork for what has become a significant focus of my career and continues to open doors for inspiring professional opportunities and growth. For me, *becoming* a Caritas Coach was a process, but *being* a Caritas Coach will be a lifelong journey.

INFORMING MY PRACTICE

Caring Science regularly informs my thinking and practice as it pertains to my presence as a leader, as well as my role as a physician for hospitalized children. What I have gained most from Caring Science is a constant self-awareness. Of course, I am not infallible. But when I do stumble, I catch myself and do what I can to amend my actions—sometimes even asking for a "do-over" when things don't go as planned.

One day, during rounds, I told a patient's family that the patient would be discharged later that day. The patient's mother became angry and withdrawn. It was evident that she was not comfortable or in agreement with this plan. My team and I walked away from this interaction feeling unsettled. After a moment, I stopped. "You know what?" I said. "We can do better than that." I took the supervising resident and intern back to the bedside and asked for another conversation with the patient's mother. Then, rather than feel defensive and guarded, frustrated by her communication style, I allowed myself to feel compassion for her experience, listened with authenticity, allowed her to express her concerns, and worked with her to devise a plan that was more agreeable for all. Not only was this an opportunity to care more authentically for a patient and family, it was a chance to model humility and self-awareness for my trainees.

Caring Science also informs my thinking and practice in my leadership role, allowing me to speak the truth with authenticity. This doesn't always make me everyone's favorite person. But it does allow for open dialogue and for the airing of important perspectives. To make a difference we must be able to speak our truth—even if it's not always well received. Culture can't change if we remain silent. This may mean conveying the perspectives of front-line staff to higher-level leaders who may be unaware of dynamics affecting patient care and experience. Indeed, speaking up on behalf of others is an important way to contribute to a caritas community. For example, after watching a patient's mother subject one of our interns to daily verbal abuse, I helped to assemble a multidisciplinary response team to support members of our staff in dealing with challenging families. I've also worked alongside my colleagues to build programs to provide debriefings for staff after emotionally difficult events such as the death of a patient. When I see suffering among caregivers through the lens of Caring Science, I am compelled to provide support and design programs to help alleviate at least some of the pain.

Creating Spirit-to-Spirit Connections

Watson writes of transpersonal caring as it relates to caritas consciousness in *Nursing: The Philosophy and Science of Caring*: "It includes perceptions and what I would call the 'phenomenal field'—the subjective and intersubjective meanings of both participants." Watson goes on to describe interconnection, referring to "higher levels of consciousness" and "transcending conventional outcomes of curing alone" (2008, p. 79).

Practicing medicine, especially pediatrics, requires one to be perceptive and to hone intuition. Sometimes this means trusting a "gut feeling" when making a diagnosis. Other times it allows for a connection with a patient or parent on a deeper emotional level. Allowing for this intuition resulted in a special connection with the father of one young patient of mine. The child had been diagnosed with Kawasaki disease, a condition in which the etiology is not fully understood. The child had responded well to treatment and shown excellent recovery. Still, during a discussion with the child's father, I could see fear in his eyes. Rather than continuing with my rounds, I hung back. We discussed his concerns, and I tried to reassure him about his child's good prognosis. The following morning, as we were hashing out discharge plans, the child's father gave me a hug. He tearfully thanked me for taking the time to speak with him the previous day. This moment filled me with joy. I truly identified with one of the reasons I had chosen medicine as a career: I wanted to help people, and I felt like I had made a difference. By pausing, being attuned to my intuition, and taking time for conversation and clarification, I gave this man a deeper level of healing and care. I frequently reflect on and draw energy from this caring experience as I ponder my own values and purpose.

Watson states, "The notion of transpersonal invites full loving-kindness and equanimity of one's presence in the moment, with an understanding that a significant caring moment can be a turning point in one's life." She goes on to describe how an "authentic spirit-to-spirit connection" can allow us to open our heart and head to what is truly emerging (Watson, 2008, p. 79). This can be applied in countless ways. For me it might be the most poignant message of Caring Science. It isn't about being flawless; it is about taking the opportunity in any moment, any interaction, to pause, reflect, connect, and assess—to ask myself, is this how I want to be? It is having self-compassion, forgiving myself and others, maybe making a course correction or taking a do-over, and working to be closer to the open-hearted, authentic, caring individual I strive to be.

PRACTICING MINDFULNESS

Caring literacy as a guiding principle allows for an ongoing cycle of perception, self-awareness, self-compassion, and growth. Thinking about practicing in the healthcare environment not as a set of actions but as a way of being inspires me to remain aware of the caritas practices and to remind myself and others about our impact on the healing environment.

One of the first Caring Science principles I learned about comes from the Halldorsdottir model, discussed by Watson (2008, p. 85). This model describes the continuum of caring from the patient's perspective, from biogenic (life-giving) to biocidic (life-destroying). Although presented by Watson as it relates to nurse-patient relationships, the model applies to anyone working in healthcare. Knowing my actions and emotions have an effect on the caring environment—and that this effect can be either healing or toxic—I try to be constantly aware of the impact I am making.

I apply these concepts in my professional sphere by bringing intentionality to my work. As a hospitalist inpatient attending, I spend a week at a time caring for a group of patients and their families and also supervising a team of trainees. At the start of each week I set an intention for how I want the week to go. This starts with self-awareness around how I show up each day. Do I bring a sense of compassion and positivity? Am I present with each patient encounter? Do I allow for authentic connection and understanding, not only of medical conditions and concerns but of the entire experience of the patient and family? What kind of role model am I being as a teacher and an attending physician? What skills do I teach trainees about their resilience and how best to approach their roles as physicians or healthcare practitioners?

I have tried different methods, but I find that the more specific I am with this intentionality, the better the effect. Recently, my intention was to foster happiness among my patients and families by promoting well-being among my team of students and residents. My plan was to implement a daily resilience practice. On one day, I had everyone share one good thing that had happened to them recently. On another day we paused by a window during rounds to reflect on the view of the Rocky Mountains outside. On yet another day I sent them all to lunch and for a walk outside while I held their phones and pagers. The ripple effect this had on the team was remarkable. Their energy seemed higher, trainees seemed to have brighter affects, and patients received excellent care. Thanks to these effects—along with the impact of one outstanding supervising resident who made a practice of thanking everyone with authenticity for every task they did—I experienced one of the most positive attending weeks I have had in my 10 years as a hospitalist. Although circumstances vary, this was an excellent lesson for me on how an emphasis on our way of *being* can affect our way of *doing*.

Self-awareness and reflection are paramount to providing authentic care as a physician and as a leader. Setting the intention to be present and compassionate in every patient interaction means remaining aware of what state of being I bring to each experience. Understanding my emotional, spiritual, intellectual, and cognitive state when interacting with colleagues and making medical decisions is essential to my remaining attentive during each encounter. Throughout each day I stay mindful of how I am coming across and take time to reflect.

Sometimes I recognize opportunities to do things differently. When I reflect on moments in which I didn't fully embody the caritas literacies or I realize I could have handled a situation better,

I acknowledge them, try to make them teachable moments, and certainly revisit them with colleagues, patients, and families when given the chance. It is easy to become defensive, especially when the stress and fatigue that stems from caring for many sick children and their families take their toll. But I'm proud when I seize an opportunity to show humility and vulnerability and seek forgiveness from those who may not have seen me at my best.

One experience stands out, in which I realized my own biases were contributing to my impatience and interfering with my ability to communicate optimally with a patient's family. As the medical director of the unit, I receive all patient complaints. One day, I received a complaint from one family about me. I immediately felt defensive. But through self-awareness and reflection I was able to acknowledge this family's complaint. Although I was extremely busy, I met with the family to let them vent their concerns. By being present and truly listening I was able to hear the family and address their frustrations. Wishing these moments didn't happen does not make it so. I instead rely on Caring Science strategies to handle them to the best of my abilities, with intention and compassion.

FINAL REFLECTIONS

My caritas journey is rooted in Caritas Process 1: "Practicing loving-kindness and equanimity for self and other" (Watson, 2008, p. 47). In my journey toward self-healing and in practicing loving-kindness toward myself, becoming a Caritas Coach enabled me to connect with my passion and calling of caring for caregivers—in other words, healing the healers. This work has supported my personal and professional growth, my consciousness of the kind of physician and colleague I aspire to be, and my efforts to support resilience and well-being for healthcare providers. My hope and dream is that with time, resilience and well-being for healthcare providers will be enculturated into healthcare environments everywhere.

Reference

Watson, J. (2008). *Nursing: The philosophy and science of caring* (rev. ed.). Boulder, CO: University Press of Colorado.

CARITAS LEADERSHIP: A VISION FOR THE FUTURE

REFLECTIONS OF A CARITAS COACH

-REID BYRNE, MSN, MA, CNM,
CARITAS COACH, REIKI MASTER, CMT

At the heart of Reid's caritas journey is the development of a richer understanding of the human experience and the mysteries of life. Reid shares how she learned to repattern her way of being when relating to others. This paradigm shift has led to an ongoing journey of self-discovery in which Reid engages in life at a higher level of consciousness, affecting the meaning of her life in profound ways.

REID'S CARITAS JOURNEY

I have always been inclined to explore the mystical and metaphysical. I often wonder, was this how caritas found me? Or did I seek caritas because I felt thirsty, and I needed to refill my cup? In truth, I think it was a bit of both—a serendipitous merging of seeking and finding. Either way, like anyone drawn to Caring Science, I was brought to it by something bigger than myself.

When I think about caritas, it's a little bit like hearing a siren's song. I feel helpless to resist. I want to immerse myself in it, but it is incredibly hot and blindingly bright. It is also like standing in front of a blank canvas. I want to create the masterpiece that is so clear in my inner vision. But I know how arduous it will be to attend to every detail while at the same time letting go of the fear it might not turn out like the vision in my mind. It is almost painful. Nevertheless, I am compelled to let go and allow my paintbrush to fly across the canvas. Being a Caritas Coach is like this. It's a paradox. As a Caritas Coach I simultaneously feel exhilarated, inspired, inadequate, and vulnerable.

I have an incessant inner drive to do, to create, to plunge myself in the energy of sensation, emotions, and understanding. This drive is so powerful it can be a bit scary. It has peaks and valleys. As a Caritas Coach, I have worked to develop the ability to notice these things—to recognize energy within self and other and to be an active participant in its use in the world.

The Caritas Coach Education Program (CCEP) helped me develop a richer understanding of my human experience and how to dive deeper into the mysterious depths of my becoming. This can be a daunting process. Fortunately, I had like-minded peers who consistently offered guidance and support. We walked the path of becoming vulnerable and working through our fears of the shadows in our psyche. We shared a mutual calling to develop a language to describe our experiences and discern how we are all interconnected. Having grasped these universal truths, we continue our process of being and becoming Caritas Coaches and of bringing caritas into the world wherever we are called to serve.

A PROCESS OF BEING AND BECOMING

I consider myself both to *be* a Caritas Coach and perpetually in the process of *becoming* a Caritas Coach. Indeed, I believe we are all perpetually in the process of becoming—becoming more compassionate, more forgiving, more grateful, more willing to love, and more willing to actively remain in the trenches to help others heal in the front lines of life (Watson, 2005).

Being and becoming are two different experiences. *Becoming* is an action word that describes movement between potential energy to kinetic energy. With becoming there is a sense of an energetic shift. Generally, becoming is not a gentle process. It takes time and requires the repatterning and assimilation of beliefs and perspectives. In contrast, *being* implies the presence of one's awareness in the here and now. Being also includes a multidimensional experience of the here and now—beyond the physical.

Watson (2008) agrees with David Bohm, who says meaning is a form of being. How we assign meaning can change the character of being. What we choose to become aware of in the present moment can dramatically change our experiences of being, such as when nurses expand their awareness to include the patient's experience on multiple dimensions and extrapolate meaning from the patient's perspective. The nurse is an integral part of this process, and his or her experience transcends the patient/nurse interaction to create a combined experience with infinite ripples of meaning, levels of awareness, and responses. I combine Bohm's "meaning" with my understanding of multidimensional awareness and Watson's *infinite transcendence* to come to what I believe is the ultimate description of being.

The Multidimensionality of Being

Watson says that in everything we do, we contribute to and participate in the web of life, existing within the infinite transcendence of
the spirit over the physical body and beyond death. We transcend
"time, past, present, future; time before and time after the earth
plane of existence" (Watson, 2005, p. 137). Nurses must be aware
of what is happening with each patient on these multiple dimensions. This requires an ability to be completely present and vulnerable to the moment.

We may not be conscious of certain dimensions of an experience
until later. I believe we can reflect on an experience and recognize
knowledge we gained on a subconscious level. For example, you
might be completely present with a patient as you perform a physical assessment, accounting for all body systems and other required
data points. But later, when someone asks you how the patient is
doing, you might reflect on more aspects of the interaction than your
physical assessment and realize that this patient was not smiling or
joking in his or her typical way. You might also realize the patient's
family has stopped visiting as frequently. It quickly becomes clear
you have assessed only one aspect of the patient's being. From this
place of knowing, you can repattern your understanding to include
a more holistic view of the patient experience. You might interact in
a completely different way because of your ability to assess multiple
dimensions of a person's being at a specific time and place.

I also believe time travel is possible if we can free our minds to
embrace the concept of infinity. Watson (2005) agrees, positing
that we can transcend time as we travel among infinite dimensions
of being. I have experienced this myself. I practice a form of deep
meditation called shamanic journeying. Shamanic journeying is like
dreaming except one is not actually asleep. Instead, one shifts from
an ordinary state of awareness of daily activities to a *shamanic state
of consciousness*—an altered, non-ordinary state of reality accessed

through meditation, prayer, drumming, or some other trance-inducing activity.

The shamanic journey is integral to the healing practice of a shaman. The shaman gains powerful insight by moving between ordinary and non-ordinary realities and applies this knowledge toward healing endeavors. This dual sense of awareness is a useful tool to gain further insight into the present moment and to develop confidence in one's ability to perceive and move between multiple dimensions of reality. If I am only tuned into my ordinary consciousness, then I am not able to benefit from a deeper awareness of my inner self and my environment. This narrow lens of ordinary reality offers a finite perception; thus, we miss opportunities to gain greater insight and opportunities to derail the process of disease and dysfunction.

Shamanic journeying can be a powerful healing tool to bring us closer to wholeness and invites us to explore the concept of infinity in a practical way. As my discernment has developed through the years, I believe I can use my shamanic practice to transcend space and time, moving into the past or future to experience a situation or be with people or guides. Through shamanic journeying, I can play out various scenarios and responses to gain a different perspective in much the same way a nurse can reflect on a patient assessment and gain a new understanding of the patient's condition and experience. I can also repattern past events in my life by returning to the place and time where I sustained an injury or psychic damage, gaining new insights on those experiences from the wisdom I have now, and assimilating these new insights into my life in the present. This deeper awareness opens me to healing in ways I never imagined were possible.

IDENTIFYING THE "REAL"

Freeing our minds to embrace the concept of infinity is one thing. But being willing to embrace a whole other level of trust—to be vulnerable and to believe that these experiences that touch on the infinite could be "real" rather than just a dream—is another. In *Harry Potter and the Deathly Hallows,* by J. K. Rowling, the main character, Harry, is killed by the villain, Voldemort. Harry finds himself in a dimension between life and death. There, he meets and converses with the spirit of his former headmaster, Dumbledore. After their conversation, Harry decides to return to his life to continue the fight against Voldemort. Before Harry leaves this shared dimension, he asks Dumbledore about their interaction: "Is this real, or has this been happening inside my head?" Dumbledore responds, "Of course it is happening inside your head, Harry, but why on Earth should that mean that it is not real?" (Rowling, 2007, p. 723). This is the quandary of faith and doubt with which we must all contend as we open ourselves to universal energies and develop a language and study of what we cannot see but sense is present and real.

Our struggle to identify and believe what is authentic and real reminds me of the old children's story *The Velveteen Rabbit,* by Margery Williams. The story is about a toy rabbit made of stuffed velveteen belonging to a young boy. The boy rarely plays with the rabbit, preferring more sophisticated toys. For a time, the velveteen rabbit is forgotten. But eventually the boy rediscovers the rabbit, and it becomes his favorite toy. In fact, the boy loves the rabbit so much it becomes real to him. However, the velveteen rabbit is *not* real to the rabbits outside. This makes the velveteen rabbit sad. He wants to be real—*really* real. Another toy called the skin horse has told the rabbit this is possible. One day the boy contracts scarlet fever. To prevent the fever from spreading, the boy's doctor orders his toys to be burnt, including the velveteen rabbit. When this happens, the rabbit cries a tear—a *real* tear. This causes a magic fairy to recognize his inner "realness" and grant his wish to become a real rabbit.

The point of the story is that what is real and what is not is often in the eye of the beholder. The rabbit becomes real through changing perspectives—his own and those of the boy, the other toys, the fairy, and the other rabbits—and by experiencing emotions like love and loss. In this modern world where emotion often is subservient to rational thinking, defining what is real is not an intellectual exercise of ranking the realness of the toys by their nature of use over time or some other objective measurement of arbitrary worth. Rather, the emotional upheaval of love, loss, grief, time, relationship, and caring support the alchemy of becoming real. In the nursing world, we champion what is real for the patient when we say things like, "Pain is what the patient says it is." Thus, we acknowledge that pain (psychological, emotional, and/or spiritual) is subjective and dependent on the perception of the individual person. This way of being with patients is authentic and honors what is real.

The velveteen rabbit experiences the process of becoming, which involves a synergy of perceptions, creation, and destruction of ways of being with one another, and finally, an uncontrolled emotional energy that animates one's life. This takes time, requires a willingness to be vulnerable, and is a process of developing wisdom and appreciation for what is truly beautiful. Perhaps the skin horse describes it best:

> "It doesn't happen all at once," said the Skin Horse. "You become. It takes a long time. That's why it doesn't happen often to people who break easily, or have sharp edges, or who have to be carefully kept. Generally, by the time you are Real, most of your hair has been loved off, and your eyes drop out and you get loose in the joints and very shabby. But these things don't matter at all, because once you are Real you can't be ugly, except to people who don't understand" (Williams, 1922, p. 3).

An important part of becoming is setting boundaries to re-pattern our evolution—even if these boundaries go against the status quo. This is particularly important in the nursing profession. More and more, nurses take on tasks of the technological and intellectual realm over the domain of psychological, emotional, and spiritual well-being (Hills & Watson, 2011). In the effort to set boundaries to repattern our evolution, we must take care not to cut ourselves off from the catalyst that makes us real: emotion, especially as it is expressed through love. Boundaries are necessary for us to protect our ability to feel. If we do not set these boundaries, we either burn out or shut down in order to cope.

In my case, boundaries safeguard against the implosion of my emotions and strengthen my commitment to my profession and myself. Setting boundaries is not always easy for me, however. I am constantly trying to become better, wiser, and smarter in my efforts to accomplish my soul's work within my specialty as a certified nurse-midwife (CNM). Some might say I am a workaholic. I am equally driven during my personal time, constantly launching and completing projects to improve my home, my workplace, my community, and myself. I constantly struggle to set boundaries with myself. It is almost as though I believe I am not real unless I am constantly occupied, and so I continue to bite off more than I can chew. Rumination and overstimulation prevent me from creating space in my life simply to feel without commentary and without needing to do anything about my emotional state in that moment. I begin to lose the resiliency and capacity to be present and to receive the insights that open up my sense of beingness in a multidimensional reality. All I can see is the task at hand, which causes me to become separated from my family, creating suffering that I feel deeply. My pain provides immediate feedback. It is like an addiction to a familiar cycle of being but never becoming something more, different, or real on any other level. Through self-love, however, I have learned that it is kind to set limits—even when I do not want to. In these times, I need the grace to choose a different path. Setting boundaries that provide space as I struggle to be compassionate with myself is what turns me into a real person—one who can forgive myself and change my behavior. I make better choices than I used to. I am in the process of becoming.

DEVELOPING CARITAS CONSCIOUSNESS AND PRACTICING SELF-CARE

Evolving as both an individual and a healthcare practitioner requires attention to self-healing and personal growth. When we take care of our own heart, we are more capable of staying in our heart center as we deliver healing services. We are more able to evolve as agents of healing energy through our authentic presence, relationship-based care, bedside manner, research, and teaching (Watson, 2005). This skill—this caritas consciousness—must be developed in many dimensions of life.

Caritas Process 1, "Practicing loving-kindness and equanimity for self and other," is foundational to caritas consciousness. Practicing self-care means developing the skills to acknowledge my feelings and validate their authenticity and worth (Watson, 2008, p. 47). This informs my way of thinking and enables me to choose a glass-half-full approach, which in turn enables me to practice the art and science of nursing from a place of authenticity, wholeness, and compassion. As a Caritas Coach, self-care—the sacred act of honoring one's personal needs—is a core skill.

Developing the wherewithal to do this very difficult work requires us to identify self-care practices with intentionality. Watson (1999) describes intentionality as a shifting of one's energy to a higher vibration—beyond the consciousness of self to that of the higher universal consciousness. Within this universal consciousness—which exists beyond the local physical body and transcends time and space—we are all interconnected beings (Watson, 2005). As Watson explains:

> The universe is a hologram...if the part is in the whole and vice versa, if even one practitioner prepares self for caritas consciousness as the basis for professional caring practices, that one nurse is

> helping transform and affect the entire field. Imagine what it would be like if nurses collectively engaged in meditative practices to cultivate caritas consciousness. (Watson, 2008, pp. 58–59)

Intentionality connects us with universal consciousness. This differs from intention, which is a mental construct that we set to overcome obstacles to achieve specific goals (Watson, 1999). If we do not connect with this universal consciousness, which provides us access to grace and serendipity, we limit our awareness to what we think we can control or manipulate, and suffer as a result. This separation from universal consciousness invariably results in caregiver burnout (Watson, 2008). In my practice, I know I am getting fatigued when I feel anxiety, I cannot catch my breath, I start talking faster, or my brain feels foggy. A commitment to self-care means that I acknowledge when I start to feel this way and set boundaries to protect my space so I can recharge. In the clinical setting, everything seems pressing. But in most cases—except in dire emergencies, of course—we can take a few moments to ask ourselves what we need to do to realign ourselves. (Naturally, this requires an ability to discern what those needs are.) Depending on the level of function (or dysfunction) in your work environment, this might seem scary. You may wonder if others will understand or if they will think you are lazy or crazy or weak or [fill in the blank]. Regardless, taking steps to recharge will build your stamina, strengthen your ability to set boundaries, and develop your awareness of what is happening within and outside yourself in each moment. This awareness and inner resilience enables you to cultivate your practice of loving-kindness toward self and others by tapping into a multidimensional source of universal consciousness through intentionality.

The work of nursing can be so depleting. We must learn to connect with the loving forces within our environment and ourselves and reclaim the energy we give to others through a practice of self-care. Reflection shapes my caritas consciousness. It illuminates my path. Through reflection I consciously acknowledge lessons learned and identify when I am depleted or distracted from my path—when

I'm "falling asleep" in my life. All this serves to sustain me as I experience the light and harmony of success as well as the dark nights of the soul.

There is a brutal edge to self-awareness and reflection, however. This requires me to be honest with myself in discerning my true feelings and motivations. Meditation, prayer, yoga, and any other practice I use to calm my mind and discover my true self can easily turn into a superficial spiritual practice if I am not willing to be vulnerable to the feelings it evokes and listen to the guidance it provides.

I am not perfect. There are days when I struggle to practice self-care. But Caring Science allows me to embrace even these negative feelings without judgment. This is imparted through Caritas Process 5: "Being present to, and supportive of, the expression of positive and negative feelings as a connection with deeper spirit of self and the one-being-cared-for" (Watson, 2008, p. 101). I accept my feelings and look for the light of understanding. Having a self-care practice helps me accept myself and stay present in relationships with others, even when it is difficult. My understanding of universal consciousness, of our oneness, helps me to remain humble and to recognize I am no better or worse than anyone else.

I believe we are all energetic beings who have no beginning and no end and that what happens in one community affects all communities. I choose to believe this because it brings me peace. It enables me to connect with the humanity and spark of love in another, no matter who they are or what they have done. I choose this way of being because it brings me comfort as I work on the front lines of suffering and disease.

A Framework and Language for Caring

The 10 Caritas Processes are a framework and language for caring literacy. They provide a structured way of thinking about concepts of caring. Each Caritas Process is a unique expression of the theory of Caring Science.

Developing a framework and language to teach Caring Science is similar to setting a foundation to teach an energy healing technique like Reiki. As a Reiki master, I begin by imparting foundational knowledge about how energy flows through the body, demonstrating a basic routine of hand positions on the body, and providing practice time to explore how individuals express their energy pattern in functional and dysfunctional ways. But the practice of energy transmutation for healing involves far more than hand placement and didactic knowledge, just as Caring Science goes far beyond the 10 Caritas Processes.

For beginners, it is helpful to explore these concepts close to the shore of the intellect—for example, through workshops, classes, and books. It also helps to establish a safe space to talk about personal experiences involving energetic relationships that are difficult to explain such as empathy, precognition, and what it means to be human.

MAINTAINING PRESENCE

My work as a nurse-midwife keeps me grounded in the moment. Caring for a woman and family through pregnancy and birth captures my full attention and keeps me present. Each woman has a unique experience of pregnancy and birth with each child she carries.

Never is it more important to stay in the present moment than when a woman is having a labor contraction! If she begins to think ahead or to remember past traumatic experiences, she will no longer be present and will lose her power. As a coach, I help my patients remain present and I act as a guardian of and witness to their experience. We share this experience through our connection to the universal consciousness. The boundaries between us become blurred. This process enables me to be more sensitive to what she needs—

sometimes so much so that I can feel what she is feeling (although to a lesser extent). This shared experience opens my heart and connects me to the divine mystery.

Of course I try to be present, using my wisdom and skills to help her, but I also need to be willing to sit in a place of not knowing and to be comfortable with discomfort. When I am at peace in this space of being fully present, I can communicate on a higher level and make choices based on my intuition rather than fear. At the same time, I am called to be a guardian of the birth space and to be aware of the energies in the environment to create and maintain harmony (Fahy & Hastie, 2008). Remaining present in my heart enables me to sustain a higher energy vibration. This affects my external environment to preserve a healing and sacred space.

Here is a poem I wrote in February 2016 to describe how transpersonal caring manifests in my practice and in my life.

— THE EMBODIMENT OF SPIRIT IN BIRTH WORK—
By Reid Byrne

Birth is a time of power and vulnerability

Tears of happiness and joy

Sighs of relief and expulsion

Looks of understanding, disbelief, love, wonder, and connection

As an observer, I experience these moments rolling through me

Some lodge themselves in my memory forever

Others hold me up as I float atop the river of life

I am in awe of the power and beauty of these moments

These incredible moments reveal something so spectacular that tears erupt from my heart and stream down my face

These visions of strangers' births elicit emotions that cannot be contained

Each person is unique and brings their own spectrum of colors to the portrait of life

But together we are stronger; we lean on each other, become vulnerable
together, and channel power to move through the cycles of life

These emotions are healing, they are human, and they are real

We answer the invitation to join in a unitary field of consciousness

We connect with all life forms through compassionate understanding of the
universal experience of pain and birth

Through love we create life, love cocoons us as we develop, and love wraps us
within its invisible tendrils to carry us through all our days

I serve as a witness to the universal human experience through birth

These shared experiences are portals, an imprint these precious souls leave
behind like breadcrumbs, through which

I find my way home.

CREATING A HEALING ENVIRONMENT

One way I manifest transpersonal caring in my practice is by transmuting one form of energy into another to create a healing environment. This exemplifies Caritas Process 8: "Creating a healing environment at all levels" (Watson, 2008, p. 129). *Transmutation* is a process of changing one frequency of energy into another. Everything is made of energy, which fluctuates constantly. Part of my practice is to help nurses and healthcare workers develop an awareness of how they affect and are affected by their environment, learn how to create a more healing environment for the self and the patient, and create a culture of caring that supports this endeavor.

Florence Nightingale considered attention to the patient's environment a core competency of nursing (Jarrin, 2012; Watson, 2008). Watson expands the traditional view of environment from the carative essentials of the physical environment—privacy, comfort, noise, lighting, safety, cleanliness, etc.—to a multidimensional unitary environmental field (Watson, 2008). This environmental field includes the interaction of the nurse and the patient within the clinical context (Jarrin, 2012; Misri, Abizadeh, Sanders, & Swift, 2015).

When we acknowledge that the nurse is part of the environment, we begin to understand how we can mold the environmental field (and by extension interpersonal relationships) into one that allows for holistic compassionate care by patterning or repatterning the environment (Watson, 2008). From this deeper understanding of the environmental field, nurses can introduce caring-healing modalities such as intentional or healing touch, art, aromatherapy, visualization, etc., with increased intuition regarding patient needs. The patient then perceives the nurse's way of being as a reflection of the inner and outer environment (Jarrin, 2012; Watson, 2008).

For the nurse, becoming aware of the environmental field involves tuning into subtle energies. It requires a willingness to be vulnerable and to not know. The nurse must regard himself or herself as well as the patient as energetic vibrational fields that are part of and affect the larger whole. The nurse's mood, beliefs, and agenda affect this human-environmental field. This expands the nurse's role in the space occupied by the nurse and patient (Watson, 2008).

Breath work is an easy but powerful technique for tuning into these subtle energies, becoming present in the moment, and developing a caring-healing practice using intentionality. Through breath work, the nurse becomes attuned to his or her heartfelt and loving intentions toward the patient. From this shift into heart-centered consciousness, the nurse shapes the environment and patient-nurse experience (Watson, 2008).

I am very sensitive to energies in my environment. As a Reiki master, I have studied and developed this sensitivity so I can detect and transmute energy from one form to another. For example, when I walk into a patient room, it may feel heavy. I center myself through my breath and open myself up to my environment. I assess my outer environment—my body language, tone of voice, state of cleanliness, interactions between people, etc. I also assess my inner environment—whether I feel anxious, rushed, angry, nauseous, dizzy, sad, etc. Identifying and acknowledging one's inner and outer perceptions as real can be difficult for beginning-level practitioners, but it is necessary in order to understand and work with the energies that are present.

CREATING A CULTURE OF CARING

Culture is intangible but powerful. Hills and Watson (2011) identify several components of culture, including values, perceptions, past associations, and shared mind-sets. Members of each nursing unit have their own ways of talking and relating to each other, sharing certain assumptions, developing shortcuts for engaging with one another, and perceiving the act of caring. These ways of being are the unit's culture.

Nurses can create a culture of caring by sharing power with each other and with their patients rather than using their power against one another, and by seeing the other as a part of the larger whole. This concept reflects the unitary field of consciousness and the holographic premise of caritas consciousness. Watson (2008) purports that a single nurse can change the universe through individual acts of loving-kindness. Likewise, each nurse can create and be an expression of the unit culture by developing awareness of how he or she co-creates the environment. The work environment affects how nurses create a culture of caring (Jarrin, 2012; Hills and Watson, 2011).

As a Caritas Coach, I want to help people creatively draw the attention of nurses toward how they can deliberately co-create and influence the patient's healing environment. I also want to help people provide external reminders to nurses to redirect their awareness to the moment and mindfully engage in patient care. These frequent reminders nudge the unit culture to provide compassionate care for the patient, family members, nurses, and staff present on the unit.

Rituals and Symbols in Caring and Healing Practices

Rituals and symbols are excellent tools to remind nurses to create a healing environment and a culture of caring. These rituals and symbols arise from a creative energy that is nonlinear. Developing and using rituals and symbols is a process of claiming the energy that rises within, co-creating with it, and healing self and others through storytelling using aesthetic expression (Samuels & Rockwood-Lane, 2013).

Rituals and symbols emanate multidimensional power. For example, the symbol for Caring Science is a circle containing the words compassion, wisdom, love, and caring. Within the circle is a lotus flower cradled in leaves and lily pads that resemble hands. The circle represents infinity, the divine feminine, unity, and wholeness. The lotus flower imparts the true nature of all sentient beings and reflects how we ascend from suffering toward enlightenment, beauty, and clarity. The leaves and lily pads represent gratitude. This symbol activates ways of knowing, being, and doing in the caring process (Watson, 1999). Many of us wear this symbol as a reminder to ourselves and to provide an opportunity to share its meaning with others—to explain what Caring Science is, how it relates to authentic presence and transpersonal connection via caritas consciousness, and what it means to be a caritas nurse.

When developing rituals and symbols, I use Caritas Process 6, "Creative use of self and all ways of knowing/being/doing as part of the caring process (engaging in artistry of caring-healing practices)" (Watson, 2008, p. 107). In this way, I am able to create rituals and symbols that reflect deep and meaningful concepts and represent the enlightenment gained through our journey as spiritual beings having a human experience. The artistry comes from the symbol itself—the creativity in how I use the symbol. The intentionality of sharing this creation inspires and renews its power within others and myself.

As I write of my experience creating and sharing the energy of a ritual, symbol, or other work of art, a Navajo/Dine saying comes to mind: "Walk in beauty." When we walk in beauty, we live in coherence with the natural order of life. This involves a journey through our living moments with love and compassion in our hearts. Beauty and love exist within and around us in the form of rituals and symbols. They are among the infinite ways aesthetic works of art empower us to walk in beauty.

TRANSPERSONAL CARING RELATIONSHIPS

Caritas Process 7 reads as follows: "Engaging in genuine teaching-learning experiences within context of caring relationship—attend to whole person and subjective meaning; attempt to stay within other's frame of reference (evolve toward 'coaching' role vs. conventional imparting of information)." Interestingly, the more I understand myself, the more I can understand another person, enter his or her frame of reference, and distinguish it from my own. Attempting to stay within the other's frame of reference means that the nurse or teacher must be sensitive to the patient or student's readiness to learn and heal and must use language that is non-threatening to their core belief system (Watson, 2008, p. 125).

Meeting people where they are in their belief system and their understanding of healing is a delicate endeavor. Watson (2008) recognizes the role of the coach or teacher as a guide to enable students to find their own answers and name their own experiences, those that are real and meaningful for them. As a Caritas Coach, my job is to help others seek a deeper, multidimensional understanding of their experience. At the same time, I must recognize the boundaries between self and other to avoid projection.

Among other things, this means becoming more comfortable sharing our stories. It means finding the words to describe experiences that have altered our understanding of caring and to participate in transpersonal, caring relationships. Watson accepted the challenge to quantify caring and create a language we can use to identify key processes and behaviors that enable healing and connection within ourselves, our patients, our community, our world, and whatever might exist beyond that. Caring literacy requires some amount of intellectual process to understand. But as we become more comfortable with its concepts and language, we add our own expression, unique skills, and interpretations to the universal experience of life. This is how we bring ourselves to the communal table as healers, guides, and students of life.

Becoming a Caritas Coach has enabled me to apply this powerful energy as a lens through which to understand and articulate the human experiences I encounter each day. In simple terms, it helps me view things from a glass-half-full perspective. I can choose to see another's action as a challenge to my personal beliefs or as an opportunity for growth and understanding. When I can pause long enough to intentionally recognize what I am feeling in the moment and at the same time seek common ground, I find a sense of peace within a burgeoning storm of misunderstanding. This energy is also an activating force for change and growth, both personally and professionally.

THE SPIRAL OF EVOLUTION

Each of us is changed by every encounter we have. This results in a constant state of evolution and development. Evolution demands sacrifice—a letting go. This is difficult to recognize and even more difficult to do.

Life has taught me that evolution in personal growth operates like a spiral. First, there is the identification of emotions. I must discern what emotions I am feeling and how they are interconnected within the web of my life experiences. This process requires trust in my interpretation of my emotions, of their interconnectivity to other facets of my life, and of their contextual meaning. I believe my spirit knows what is best for me. Therefore, I remain open to the wisdom that comes through when I create sacred space to listen. Next, I must use this new awareness to make choices. Assimilating the changes that accompany these choices and the new and deeper awareness that develops usually results in some amount of tumult. Finally, I let go of my former understanding. I can then enjoy a more peaceful time—that is, until life pitches a new situation, and I must start the cycle all over again.

I continue to strive to make wiser choices based on this spiraling evolution of self-awareness and reflection. It requires courage and energy to create the sacred space to reflect, acknowledge, and recognize the changes needed to align my heart, mind, and spirit. However, when I do this with intentionality, I have always been led down the right path for me in that place and time. Because evolution occurs in a spiral, the seasons of learning are always changing as we grow. Time is a whole other dimension to our growth with which we must partner. And of course, we must let go of the idea that we can control anything at all.

THE NEED FOR CARING CURRICULUM

Through the CCEP I have learned a language and framework to name and validate the energies I experience. I have also learned to seek congruence and authenticity in how I choose to interact with my internal and external environment. This inner knowing is hard to quantify but it is a vital part of caritas.

During my training as an advanced practice nurse, I was drawn to this program because it served as a counterbalance to a nursing education system that values research, science, and rational thinking. Institutions offering nursing education struggle to offer a curriculum that conveys both the necessary intellectual and didactic knowledge of nursing and the inner knowledge that enables us to honor our hearts, to heed the call to be present with patients, and to develop the keen discernment needed to identify what each patient needs in order to be healed (not necessarily cured) and to feel like he or she is not alone (Watson, 2008; Hills & Watson, 2011).

These programs fail to balance the more masculine Western rational thinking ethos with the sacred feminine archetype that values carative (rather than curative) practice, equilibrium, and harmony. It is as if the world of academia is just as pressured by the drive for knowledge as the healthcare system is by the drive to cure disease and prevent death. This frequently forces nurses away from the "soft" skills of caring toward "hard" scientific facts. If these soft skills are covered at all, too often it is left to the end of the academic program or presented in an employee self-care program that serves as an accreditation requirement. Student nurses and practitioners alike receive the tacit message that reflecting and developing an inner knowing is not as valuable as applying the conventional scientific method to everything they do.

Nurses have long recognized the shortcomings of nursing curriculum. Watson and other scholars have identified the importance of introducing nurses (and other healthcare professionals) to a language that enables them to reflect and discuss their experiences while they are in school (Hills & Watson, 2011). In recent years many nursing schools have begun to include Caring Science as part of their vision and to incorporate it throughout their curriculum (Clark, 2016). Caring Science provides a method for well-intentioned schools to actualize their goal to develop clinically proficient nurses who provide compassionate care. It conceptualizes the patient and the practitioner as a synergistic expression of the art and science of healing.

This has not always worked, however. For example, my graduate program included curriculum that recognized the value of reflection and of a practitioner's inner knowing but devoted too little time to helping students learn the common language of caring. We end up with either superficial attempts to develop the competency of being and becoming a caring practitioner, or inconsistent instruction based on the comfort level of the instructor. Faculty need to be empowered to obtain Caring Science literacy and to create courses that incorporate concepts such as authentic presence, inner knowing, the evolution of human consciousness, healing through aesthetics and connection with one's environment, and viewing caring inquiry as a valid methodology for developing and quantifying evidence (Hills & Watson, 2011).

I truly believe these schools and healthcare systems mean well. I believe they value the philosophy of Caring Science. But our culture has a long history of valuing reason over intuition (Watson, 1999). We must fight the temptation to abandon the ground gained from Watson's work. Nursing curriculum must reflect this new paradigm to support the evolution of our healing practice. Nursing and medicine, as professions and as archetypes, must come together as equals to yield a new paradigm of understanding (Watson, 1999). For the healing profession to evolve, academic institutions, healthcare institutions, and society as a whole must honor and assist practitioners in their commitment to be and become more compassionate and more aware of how loving, heart-centered care unifies and heals all of us.

In the meantime, Caritas Coaches serve as the champions of Caring Science and as translators for caring language that combines reason, emotion, and intuition. Nurses and healthcare professionals deserve someone who understands the need to reflect, and who can help them find words to express their inner knowing and the courage to co-create a new reality. The Caritas Coach is the expert in the field to whom nurses and other healthcare professionals can turn for assistance when they want to "go with their gut" but cannot explain why.

The Caritas Coach is not an expert with special knowledge or authority. Rather, the role of the Caritas Coach is to facilitate the capacity of others to discover creative solutions for themselves and to encourage and celebrate their efforts and growth (Watson, 2008). In my role as Caritas Coach, I offer myself as a guide for nurses and other healthcare providers, patients, and family members. My role as a Caritas Coach is one of a space holder, guardian, translator, and conduit—for whatever is *being* in the present moment and whatever is in the process of becoming. I help to create a sacred space that makes room for the unknown and honors all who participate and affect this shared experience. Indeed, I took a leave of absence from my school in order to do this in an intentional way. Caring Science feeds my spirit and nurtures the calling I feel to share this perspective of caring in a way my peers and colleagues can understand.

DISCOVERING SELF AND OTHER

Self-care cultivates sensitivity to oneself and others. This is a lifelong process of growth and development. It does not stop just because I have obtained a certificate calling me a coach. In my case, I am constantly challenged to learn what self-care can be and to give myself permission to affirm my needs for nurturing. Caritas Process 3, "Cultivating one's own spiritual practices; deepening self-awareness, going beyond 'ego-self'" (Watson, 2008, p. 68), is a vital step in my own development.

Through Caring Science, I have become more aware of my personal struggle to set boundaries and maintain the discipline of self-care to cultivate my own spiritual growth. This translates into compassion for others. Modeling this behavior and helping others develop self-compassion and self-care supports the transpersonal nature of the teaching-learning experience. I feel certain the universe will provide me with even more opportunities to teach what I am learning about self-care to others.

Perhaps my most difficult struggle with self-care is recognizing my own humanity. I must learn to forgive myself when I fall into the trap of believing I need to do more, do better, or do differently. I must accept my mistakes. I must offer myself compassion when I feel vulnerable and unsure. In his book *The Four Agreements: A Practical Guide to Personal Freedom*, Don Miguel Ruiz observes that what constitutes "our best" changes moment to moment in accordance with how we feel. "Just do your best—in any circumstance in your life," he writes. "It doesn't matter if you are sick or tired, if you always do your best there is no way you can judge yourself.

And if you don't judge yourself there is no way you are going to suffer from guilt, blame, and self-punishment" (Ruiz & Mills, 1997, p. 78). If you do your best, you can always forgive yourself if your efforts do not quite measure up to expectations. Ruiz goes on to write, "Once you forgive yourself, the self-rejection in your mind is over. Self-acceptance begins, and the self-love will grow so strong that you will finally accept yourself just the way you are. That's the beginning of the free human" (Ruiz & Mills, 1997, p. 116). This is the way toward true healing.

FINAL REFLECTIONS

Caring Science is more than a new lens through which to view my world. It is more than a passive tool to adjust my perspective. It is, to borrow a phrase from *Back to the Future*, a flux capacitor that powers dimensional shifts in awareness.

This begs the question, "So what?" We still have our struggles and disappointments. We still have to get up, drink our coffee, brush our teeth, get dressed, go to work, come home, and fix dinner, not to mention deal with conflict and all the rest. But with caritas, we do it from a different perspective. Engaging with life at a higher vibration affects our environment in untold ways.

Perhaps the better question is, "Why not?" We all search for meaning on some level. We all learn from life and mature. We get to choose, at some level, the wisdom path that speaks to our hearts and fulfills us, even as it breaks through our walls and makes us uncomfortable enough to change. Why not embrace Caring Science as a path to discover meaning and help others to do the same?

Life offers us infinite opportunities and tools to support our process of becoming wise and loving beings. This wisdom is a living thing. I wish you all the best as you explore Caring Science and learn for yourself what it means to be and become a Caritas Coach.

REFERENCES

Clark, C. S. (2016). Watson's human caring theory: Pertinent transpersonal and humanities concepts for educators. *Humanities, 5*(2), 21. doi:10.3390/h5020021

Fahy, K., & Hastie, C. R. (2008). Midwifery guardianship: Reclaiming the sacred in birth. In K. Fahy, M. Foureur, & C. Hastie (Eds.), *Birth territory and midwifery guardianship: Theory for practice, education, and research* (pp. 21–37). Edinburgh, NY: Books for Midwives Press.

Hills, M., & Watson, J. (2011). *Creating a caring science curriculum: An emancipatory pedagogy for nursing.* New York, NY: Springer Publishing Co.

Jarrin, O. F. (2012). The integrality of situated caring in nursing and the environment. *Advances in Nursing Science, 35*(1), 14–24. doi:10.1097/ANS.0b013e3182433b89

Misri, S., Abizadeh, J., Sanders, S., & Swift, E. (2015). Perinatal generalized anxiety disorder: Assessment and treatment. *Journal of Women's Health, 24*(9), 762–770. doi:10.1089/jwh.2014.5150

Rowling, J. K. (2007). *Harry Potter and the deathly hallows.* London, UK: Bloomsbury Publishing.

Ruiz, D. M., & Mills, J. (1997). *The four agreements: A practical guide to personal freedom.* San Rafael, CA: Amber-Allen Publishing.

Samuels, M., & Rockwood-Lane, M. (2013). *Healing with the arts: A 12-week program to heal yourself and your community.* New York, NY: Atria Books.

Watson, J. (1999). *Postmodern nursing and beyond.* London, UK: Churchill Livingstone.

Watson, J. (2005). *Caring science as sacred science.* Philadelphia, PA: F. A. Davis Co.

Watson, J. (2008). *Nursing: The philosophy and science of caring* (rev. ed.). Boulder, CO: University Press of Colorado.

Williams, M. (1922). *The velveteen rabbit.* New York, NY: George H. Doran Company.

A Global Paradigm Shift for the Caritas Coach

–William Rosa, MS, RN, LMT, AHN-BC,
AGPCNP-BC, CCRN-CMC, Caritas Coach

In this chapter, Billy explores the global vision for caritas and for nursing's unique contributions to human health and healing environments around the world. This vision begins with each nurse's own interpersonal evolution toward being, becoming, doing, and knowing. Billy advocates a "strategic and systematic approach to human engagement and human-centered care" with Caring Science as its foundation and a new paradigm for world health.

BILLY'S CARITAS JOURNEY

In its nearly 40 years of scholarly advancement and metaphysical exploration, human Caring Science has held one belief as central and paramount: We, as human beings and as the sacred vessels of embodied spirit, are inherently interconnected through a fragile yet unbreakable web of caritas. This knowledge is a human right that seeks to remind all men, women, and children that we are part of a shared humanity—one that acknowledges, respects, and honors our uniquely evolving experiences and narratives. But this awareness carries with it an undeniable responsibility: a universal task to shift the current paradigm of separation and ego toward one of wholeness and humility; to embrace peace and peaceful practices; and to create infrastructures that promote justice, equality, and safe, inclusive environments for human flourishing.

As the keystone of Caring Science, caritas is also a primary factor in the future of planetary health and well-being. The deliberate engagement of a caritas framework has the power to transform worldviews and universal outcomes that will determine our survival—all of us. It has the potential to create unified transnational partnerships, end ongoing threats of global violence and destruction, support the realization of equality among all people and populations, and preserve nature and its resources, which are quickly being depleted worldwide. Although its conscious use carries with it great promise, an unconscious disengagement from the ethics and values of caritas has equally significant—albeit disturbing—implications. For when we forget this foundation—this sacred truth that we are one—human caring and its effects on the countless faces of the global village become just another theoretical concept without a forum for practical application.

This ancient knowledge is the substance of nursing's unique contributions to human betterment and the moral foundation of human caring that continues to awe and inspire us. Integrating this principle of caritas as a lived ethic requires a global paradigm shift that starts with our personal-professional commitment to create healing environments at all levels within, among, and between all peoples.

THE ART AND SCIENCE OF NURSE COACHING

One must understand what coaching is to differentiate it from being and becoming a Caritas Coach. For myself, the word coaching seems somewhat elementary for the delicate spirit work that is caritas. And yet, the word coaching carries with it all the implications of progress, growth, evolution, and unity suggested by a human-caring paradigm.

The art and science of nurse coaching implies a host of literacies, scopes of practice, and core values that guide personal-professional development and lead to measurable outcomes (Dossey, Luck, & Schaub, 2014). It is "a systematic and skilled process grounded in scholarly, evidence-based professional nursing practice" and "support[s]...the client's healing process as it manifests in body-mindspirit" (Dossey & Luck, 2016, p. 502). Nurse coaching as both a tool and a premise for self-other engagement promotes an environment of safety and expression where the experiences of all involved are honored as valid and vital to the integrity of the whole.

For me, being a Caritas Coach takes these principles to the next level of mind and heart consciousness, where tools and systematic approaches are humanized through the dynamic flow of relationship-based engagement. A Caritas Coach invests in the interpersonal evolution of self and other, commits to this shared experience by building and developing caring relationships, and takes accountability for his or her role in the global realities emerging all around us (Rosa, 2016a). Being, in this context, is about action: demonstrating caritas through the co-creation of compassionate partnerships with others. It is not about theory or concepts; it is about experiential wisdom and applied ethics. It is about practicing the values and employing the knowledge. It is about quite literally being the change.

Becoming a Caritas Coach is about the journey—always maintaining a heightened and more global perspective on one's intentionality, goals, successes, failures, and purpose. Note, however, that becoming is not the same as achieving. We don't achieve Caritas

Coach-hood; we become and are in continually emerging relationship with the ideals represented by the title of Caritas Coach. This happens only when we commit to a life and professional covenant that reflects caritas values and ideals. Becoming is really about striving, a concept that reminds us that the human being's primary struggle is to return to one's spiritual essence (i.e., the real self) and become more god-like in the process (Watson, 2012).

INTENTIONAL ACTION

Caring Science as a paradigm and way of being, becoming, doing, and knowing is a radical notion. It suggests an overhauling of bureaucratic constraints and of obsolete paternalistic systems that lead to dehumanized healthcare and the devaluation of nursing. It is not a "soft" concept or "gentle" paradigm, but a sturdy, strategic, and systematic approach to human engagement and human-centered care. It brings up necessary and urgent questions about who we are, what we do, and how and why we do it.

Some time ago, I wrote the following:

> Patients stand before us with rich life histories and future possibilities that often present in the context of vulnerability and suffering; the question then becomes, who are we not to care? ... Who are we if not the protectors, advocates, and givers of precious human caring? ... How are we to be in this world as mentors, teachers, role models, and caring-healing practitioners if not literate in a science of human caring? Are we to abbreviate our endless disciplinary potential to become technicians and skilled attendants? (Rosa, 2014a, p. 265)

I went on to state that indeed it is unethical not to care. Caring Science shifts the global paradigm not only with what it suggests, but also with what is suggested by its absence. A world without human caring is just that: a care-less place. What disparities, in-justices, and inequalities would take root in such a reality? What human rights and sacred truths would be stripped? Caring isn't a choice. For me, caring is a moral imperative. It is a must.

Although Caring Science is a prominent theory and ever-expand-ing ontological portal (Watson, 2008; Davidson, Ray, & Turkel, 2011; Smith, Turkel, & Wolf, 2012; Sitzman & Watson, 2016), it is known, thrives, and comes to life through intentional action. It sim-ply does not exist without evidence of its expression between people. All the countless potentials and possibilities of Caring Science fail if they are lost in the theory-practice gap. This is my daily reminder as a Caritas Coach: If I don't show up as the caring person I think I am or hope to be, then I have been a demonstration of the opposite—an example of what it is not to care.

TRUSTING AND INTIMATE RELATIONSHIPS

As I sat down to write this chapter, I received a message from a col-league that a patient I'd been caring for during the previous 3 weeks had passed away. The patient, a 51-year-old man named Jack, had been recently diagnosed with an extremely aggressive and widely metastatic esophageal cancer. Jack was an adventurous spirit who loved his life in Hawaii, traveled and saw the world, was deeply fond of his brother, and was what he called a "closet Buddhist."

Over the 20 or so days of our relationship, Jack repeated again and again that he was not afraid to die. He was, however, afraid to suffer. Jack quickly lost control of his environment and physical bearings. His breathing became more labored, his thoughts more erratic, and his demeanor increasingly despondent. On the last day I saw him, he was verbally unresponsive. I stood at his bedside and promised him that he would not suffer. I was able to keep that promise—a rare thing of beauty in modern healthcare. According to my colleague, Jack had died comfortably.

I am forever changed by knowing Jack. And I know our relationship is not over. It will continue to evolve—and not just because his brother will think of me and the support and care I provided when he remembers Jack's final days. I am confident the moments Jack and I shared together are alive and vibrating, with implications for my own healing and well-being, and for the healing and well-being of those who witnessed and shared in the short-lived trust and intimacy of our relationship.

That awareness and presence is what it means to live the transpersonal: the knowledge and belief that who I am and the caring service delivered through me is not of or about me. Rather, the healing that needs expression in a given moment takes advantage of my willingness to be an available vessel for its manifestation.

The transpersonal caring relationship I shared with Jack existed before I ever met him. It started when I saw his name on my patient list and created an intention for what our encounter would become. It grew each day through our moments together, our words exchanged, and his vulnerabilities held and honored. And it continues to mature as I reflect and grieve his passing with compassion. He will be with me forever, and I with him. That is the power of a conscious, healing, caring, transpersonal relationship.

TOWARD CARITAS LITERACY

Since graduating from the Caritas Coach Education Program (CCEP), I have consistently integrated Caring Science literature in my publications and educational endeavors with a goal to increase caritas literacy for colleagues and the profession at large. By consistently promoting Caring Science as the foundational ethic and ethos of nursing, I seek to broaden the scope of its application to a diverse set of topics—from global health and global nursing (Rosa, 2017), to effective communication and evolutionary approaches to leadership (Rosa & Santos, 2016; Rosa, 2016b), to humanistic end-of-life care and conscious dying practices (Rosa, 2014b; Rosa & Estes, 2016; Rosa, Estes, & Watson, 2017).

As we continue to develop as Caritas Coaches and human-caring advocates, we must align our work with representative organizations, scopes of practice, and caring, human-centered literacies that reflect nursing's greater altruistic purpose. This helps to define our intraprofessional identity and serves as a springboard for higher planes of caritas consciousness and a unified planetary existence.

Dossey et al. (2013) have established competencies for the professional nurse coach. This discussion hopes to drive the development of practice standards and, therefore, an emerging level of caritas literacy specifically designed for the Caritas Coach beyond nursing, beyond health, and toward a whole-person/whole-people, planetary paradigm. I suggest deepening caritas work in a way that supports the American Nurses Association (ANA, 2015a) standards of practice and professional performance, which are informed by the organization's code of ethics (ANA, 2015b), through the creation of literacies, as follows:

- Connect to self and intention before engaging with another.

- Engage with compassion and reverence for a whole-person approach to caring.

- Create environments that allow another's self-discovery to be fully expressed and honored.

- Promote acceptance of and respect for another's vulnerability, joy, grief, success, failure, and inner knowing.

- Provide empathic support for another's self-directed agency.

- Develop collaborative relationships where co-creation is free to guide and inspire positive change.

- Employ a caritas consciousness in all coaching interactions with another.

- Remain aware of local, global, and universal implications during coaching work.

- Stay heart-centered before, during, and after time with another to ensure self-care and healing environments for all.

- Celebrate the individual expression of another while remaining true to personal ethics and values.

- Acknowledge the unique characteristics of another as strengths for personal growth and development.

- Engage others with caritas as a starting and ending point of ethical engagement.

- Demonstrate caring as a way of honoring shared humanity and the inherent spirit nature of all.

- Practice loving-kindness for human beings, the environment, all species, and the planet at large.

- Invite all ways of knowing to understand and partner with another.

- Be flexible and adaptive in building self-other partnerships for improved understanding and knowledge.

These literacies are only a starting point for future conversations about an increased transparency and visibility of Caritas Coaching in professional nursing and in the service of human healing and wholeness. These literacies are a reflection of my personal-professional development in applying a caritas consciousness to my work as a nurse and Caritas Coach.

IMMERSION IN THE SUSTENANCE OF SELF

The endless journey into my being, toward the knowing of my fullest self and spirit, deeply and profoundly excites me. It has become my primary motivation to experience life to its fullest, to push myself past limiting definitions and beyond static patterns and comfort zones, to embrace my vulnerability and imperfection as a part of this whole and perfect being. It isn't always easy but I'm getting there. Caring Science invites us to know who we really are, beyond professional titles and personal accomplishments, toward a more inclusive understanding of shared humanity and inherent belonging to the spiritual collective. It asks us to be loving, kind, and compassionate to self and other, and to become aware of the places and spaces that need our caring attention.

Reflective practice is a cornerstone of my personal-professional life. It grants me the opportunity to make sense of the noise and grow into the stillness of who I really am. Self-reflection is a requisite of the Caritas Coach, not only as a developed skill but also as a practice of loving-kindness toward self. It requires tenderness, empathy, and the courage to engage in fearless moral exploration.

Final Reflections

The global paradigm shift implied by caritas and the work of Caritas Coaching goes beyond the current content and purpose of nursing curricula and professional nurse coach standards. Caring Science offers just one way to bring our unique and authentic selves to the sacred work of nursing and human healing in systems that are still guided and overly constrained by inhumane policies and strict standards. Caritas Coaching is a way to humanize and actualize the ideals of Caring Science and the ethical values promoted by Florence Nightingale.

Ultimately, Caritas Coaching is about our ability as leaders, advocates, professionals, guides, and human beings to accept and celebrate the wholeness of life—both the light and the shadows. We have a responsibility to embrace not only equanimity in the face of what comes our way, but also the compassionate loving-kindness that will reinforce peace, inclusiveness, and social justice for all.

Caritas starts with honoring the day, with all it brings, and the people who coexist in our world, and all they contribute to our experience on Earth. It starts with acknowledging that our experience and time here with each other go beyond anything we will ever be able to fully articulate, and yet there is a holiness and universality that constantly yearns to be seen. As we move forward in caritas, it is our responsibility to share this truth with those we know and serve.

In closing, I share the words of my dear friend Elizabeth Anne Jones—words of caritas—words that move us toward the global paradigm shift of universal love that is so needed in our times.

Thank you for this day...

My blessings, my pain, my joy.

Bless all my family,

Bless all my friends.

Bless all the people I know,

Bless all the people I don't know.

Bless all the people I will know,

Bless all the people I will never know.

Bless all life on this earth and those who have gone.

Be in my thoughts, my actions, my words,

My deeds, my intentions, my livelihood,

My mindfulness, my concentration.

Help me be the change for peace, love, compassion, and light,

And may all beings be filled with loving kindness.

Namaste.

REFERENCES

American Nurses Association (ANA). (2015a). Nursing scope and standards of practice (3rd ed.). Silver Spring, MD: Author.

American Nurses Association (ANA). (2015b). Code of ethics for nurses with interpretive statements. Silver Spring, MD: Author.

Davidson, A. W., Ray, M. A., & Turkel, M. C. (2011). Nursing, caring, and complexity science: For human-environment well-being. New York, NY: Springer Publishing Co.

Dossey, B. M., Hess, D. R., Southard, M. E., Luck, S., Schaub, B. G., & Bark, L. (2013). The art & science of nursing coaching: The provider's guide to coaching scope and competencies. Silver Spring, MD: American Nurses Association.

Dossey, B. M., & Luck, S. (2016). Nurse coaching. In B. M. Dossey & L. Keegan (Eds.), Holistic nursing: A handbook for practice (7th ed., pp. 501–511). Burlington, MA: Jones & Bartlett Learning.

Dossey, B. M., Luck, S., & Schaub, B. G. (2014). Nurse coaching: Integrative approaches for health and wellbeing. Surfside, FL: International Nurse Coach Association.

Rosa, W. (2014a). Letter to the editor: It is unethical not to care. Nursing Science Quarterly, 27(3), 265–266.

Rosa, W. (2014b). Conscious dying and cultural emergence: Reflective systems inventory for the collective processes of global healing. Beginnings, 34(5), 20–22.

Rosa, W. (2016a). Infusing nurse coaching with moral imagination: The fiber of interconnectedness. Beginnings, 36(2), 14–16.

Rosa, W. (2016b). Nurses as leaders: Evolutionary visions of leadership. New York, NY: Springer Publishing Co.

Rosa, W. (2017). A new era in global health: Nursing and the United Nations 2030 agenda for sustainable development. New York, NY: Springer Publishing Co.

Rosa, W., & Estes, T. (2016). What end-of-life care needs now: An emerging praxis of the sacred and subtle. Advances in Nursing Science, 39(4), 333–345.

Rosa, W., Estes, T., & Watson, J. (2017). Caring science conscious dying: An emerging meta-paradigm. Nursing Science Quarterly, 30(1), 58–64.

Rosa, W., & Santos, S. (2016). Introduction of the engaged feedback reflective inventory in a preceptor training program. Journal for Nurses in Professional Development, 32(4), E1–E7.

Sitzman, K., & Watson, J. (2016). Watson's caring in the digital world: A guide for caring when interacting, teaching, and learning in cyberspace. New York, NY: Springer Publishing Co.

Smith, M. C., Turkel, M. C., & Wolf, Z. R. (2012). Caring in nursing classics: An essential resource. New York, NY: Springer Publishing Co.

Watson, J. (2008). Nursing: The philosophy and science of caring (rev. ed.). Boulder, CO: University Press of Colorado.

Watson, J. (2012). Human caring science: A theory of nursing (2nd ed.). Burlington, MA: Jones & Bartlett Learning.

THE JOURNEY
FORWARD

The Ever-Evolving, Introspective, and Morally Active Life of a Caritas Coach

–Sara Horton-Deutsch, PhD, RN, FAAN, ANEF, Caritas Coach

As the stories in this book attest, a Caritas Coach is one with an ever-evolving way of being, knowing, becoming, and doing. Through deep exploration of the theory, ethic, and praxis of Caring Science, each of the Caritas Coaches who shared their stories in this book developed their own ethical and moral foundation for living through love, care, and healing of self and other. The stories also serve as a guide to a way of life grounded in Caring Science.

Whether in educational or clinical practice settings or in formal or informal leadership roles, Caritas Coaches are empowered to find and use their authentic self and unique voice and language for the promotion of health and healing for all. Through this continuous process of being and becoming, Caritas Coaches help to co-create more biogenic environments by practicing the tenets of Caring Science—sharing their values of loving-kindness, equanimity, compassion, respect, and honor for self and other.

This final chapter of the book synthesizes and extends contributors' reflections of being and becoming, and offers integral theory and emancipatory nursing praxis as a way to further advance our capacity for reflective thinking and acting—and the cultivation of an informed moral praxis.

BEING AND BECOMING A CARITAS COACH

The stories in this text give readers a glimpse into the paths of discovery of several Caritas Coaches. Throughout each account, several themes emerged including: finding their inner voice, learning to trust themselves to grow personally and professionally, and expanding their ways of knowing and doing. By engaging in creative processes drawn from the arts and humanities, they learned new ways to express their inner world, and ultimately the outer world, by connecting and relating more genuinely with others. They learned how to be responsive, thoughtful, and attuned to themselves and others, enabling them to authentically listen to another person's story.

Being and becoming more intentional and imaginative—in practice, teaching, and leading—models humanistic-altruistic values for self and other. This way of being and becoming takes more energy than just showing up for a day of work. Choosing not just what to do each day at work but *how* to work means choosing to care, love, and heal. As the stories attest, the rewards are vast, diverse, and meaningful—by staying connected to caritas literacy and to what matters most, personal and professional lives become less separate. Rather, these different life roles become synergistic. Threaded throughout the stories are examples of authentic human connections rooted in genuine relatedness.

Continuously guided by the 10 Caritas Processes, contributors engage in practices of caring that add value and meaning to each moment of the day. The emphasis on *how* as much as *what* directs the doing and evolves into becoming. For example, pausing to breathe and center before entering a patient's hospital room prepares the practitioner to be authentically present for that patient. This simple practice transforms *doing* to a way of *being* and transforms tasks into reverent acts of care and compassion. The simple task of giving a patient a glass of water can transform into a human-to-human connection if the practitioner looks into the patient's eyes, fully sees the patient, touches the patient's mind, body, and spirit, and sustains human dignity. These caring-healing practices add only seconds to one's day but immeasurable value to the life of self and other. They transform *being* into an ever-evolving *becoming*, where all vicissitudes of humanity and the human experience are welcomed and attended to, as we evolve toward deeper levels of consciousness (Watson, 2008).

Caritas practitioners nurture themselves as they evolve by integrating all ways of knowing. This further supports the development of unitary caritas consciousness (by doing as an *inner* practice of expanding awareness through reflection) and of caritas literacy (by doing as an *outer* practice of informed moral praxis). Any reflective professional engaged in caring, healing, and health is ethically obligated to pursue this level of evolved being, knowing, becoming, and doing in the world (Watson & Horton-Deutsch, 2018).

THE DEVELOPMENT OF INTEGRAL CONSCIOUSNESS

Those who enter the Caritas Coach program often recognize the need for balance, equanimity, and enhanced self-care practices in their lives. Some have contemplated leaving their professions, feeling depleted of the ability to care or give. Others have experienced health crises that required learning new self-care practices or brought a change in perspective. Still others yearn for something more and are searching for a way to have more balance and equanimity in their personal and professional lives.

Many of the narratives in this book demonstrate the development of the use of integral theory (described in the following section) and the incorporation of all ways of knowing, an approach consistent with the inclusive nature of Caring Science. Participants in the program became aware of their personal experiences through consideration of their thoughts, feelings, emotions, and bodily sensations; and through critical reflection that enabled them to develop a deeper understanding of self and other. This is consistent with the work of philosopher-scientist-practitioner Ken Wilber, who has advanced the integrally informed approach toward being and doing in the world (2000, 2001, 2005, 2007).

Wilber identifies four major perspectives or dimensions of awareness to describe a person's being in the world. The integral perspective is relayed using the acronym AQAL (All Quadrants All Levels). Figure 21.1 shows the AQAL model in picture form. It can be described as follows:

- The upper-left (UL) quadrant represents an individual's interior thoughts, feelings, emotions, and intentions—the "I" space.

- The lower-left (LL) quadrant is the collective interior. It represents the individual's relationships and culture, and the meaning the individual shares with others—the "we" space.

- The upper-right (UR) quadrant is the individual's exterior, including his or her physical body, behaviors, and actions—the "it" space.

- The lower-right (LR) quadrant is the collective exterior, including the individual's environment and social structures—the "its" space.

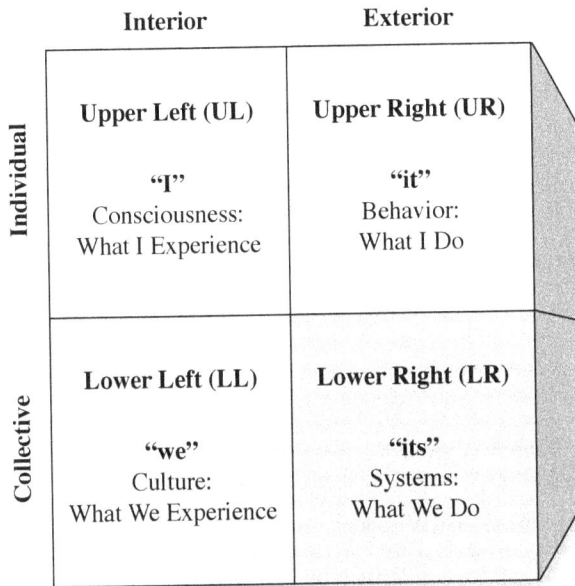

FIGURE 21.1   THE FOUR QUADRANTS OF THE AQAL MODEL.

These quadrants represent four perspectives of awareness, or four ways of knowing:

- To gain perspective from the point of the upper-left quadrant (I), one explores through journaling, mindfulness practices, reflection, meditation, and phenomenology. This self-knowledge influences how one sees the world and influences how one practices and relates to others.

- Gaining perspective from the point of the lower-left quadrant (we) involves being with another. The feeling of *we* in a relationship is fostered through understanding, reflective dialogue with others, storytelling, and/or debate.

- The upper-right quadrant (it) represents how one gains perspective from objective meaning. This is the bio-behavioral aspect of the individual—what one can see, hear, touch, taste, or smell. One can measure this *it* through empirical means of observation from the outside in—surveys, examination of documentation, representative samples, etc.

- The lower-right quadrant (its) offers perspective on social-political systems. It includes the environment, ecology, and social systems such as schools and government. One gains perspectives on the *its* quadrant by understanding interacting systems that focus on sustainability and ecology.

Integral theory supports caritas consciousness by challenging the practitioner to be aware of the four dimensions in an intentional way. Appreciating each quadrant helps us to see the bigger picture. It provides alternative ways of understanding and investigating phenomena while appreciating and honoring multiple perspectives.

Beyond the four quadrants, the integral framework includes several other elements: levels, lines, states, and types. These can be explored through Wilber's original work (2000, 2001, 2005, 2007) or through the disciplinary lens of nursing (Pesut, 2017; Pesut, Sherwood, & Horton-Deutsch, 2017).

For our purposes the key is to appreciate how to continue to expand knowing and consciousness. Today, much of healthcare education focuses on *it* knowing through mastery of empirical knowledge, tasks, and skills. Caring Science encourages us to balance this way of knowing with the other three quadrants, beginning with knowing self (I), then relating to others (we), and finally understanding and appreciating community and environments (its).

Doing as an Inner Practice of Expanding Awareness

Through the narratives in this book, contributors convey a view of human life lived reflectively—attending to and honoring self while simultaneously staying in connection with other. Being in the world in this way takes courage and emotional stamina. It requires not only presence but also the ability to listen and learn, to engage authentically with others, and to use caring language that gives voice to the greater good of humanity.

Reflecting on self is represented by the upper-left quadrant of integral theory (refer to Figure 21.1). It calls us to examine prior beliefs and assumptions and their implications. The exploration of experiences, and analysis of thoughts and feelings, informs learning. It involves a transformation in thinking that leads to action. Reflective activities such as meditation and journaling foster open-mindedness, whole-heartedness, and a sense of responsibility in facing consequences (Dewey, 1933). From a Caring Science perspective, reflective practice guides us to honor another's uniqueness and to sustain his or her human dignity.

In Western healthcare systems and academic settings, which focus almost exclusively on evidence-based practices and empirical views of measuring the world, Caritas Coaches reconnect to the value of inner knowing. There is value in simultaneously connecting inner and outer worlds, self and other. As a form of practice-based evidence, these narratives demonstrate the value of a life lived reflectively, in connection with others, and in finding meaning.

Caritas consciousness as an inner practice of expanding awareness through reflection involves being aware of the energy and vibration that come from caring and love. It manifests through being and becoming in the caring moment, positively affecting the environment. It is a reflective, authentic, and conscious practice of intentionally directing loving presence. It is nurtured by practicing loving-kindness and equanimity toward self and other. As described in the narratives in this text, caritas consciousness has enabled contributors to see and do things differently. By holding caring-healing or more loving consciousness, they could extend different messages, affecting the subtle energetic environment and spreading healing, kindness, forgiveness, and equanimity. Through this process, practitioners become the caritas field.

DOING AS AN OUTER PRACTICE OF INFORMED MORAL PRAXIS

Development of higher-level *inner* consciousness requires a demonstration of higher-level *outer* consciousness in the world, expressed through language. Through a higher level of consciousness, Caritas Coaches learn to thoughtfully use their voices to advocate for all people (patients, students, staff, colleagues, etc.), themselves, and systems. They see and demonstrate the value of flexibility, trust, and, most importantly, the need for connection. They seek creative solutions for the healthcare services people want while honoring diversity, equity, and inclusion. Caritas Coaches evolve their expectation of healthcare and how it can work through genuine collaboration and care for one another.

Like caritas consciousness, caritas literacy is nurtured through an appreciation for and integration of all ways of knowing. Both are "a special way of being, a loving, caring and compassionate human being, becoming and evolving to be more caring, kind, and compassionate with self, others, and all living things" (Watson, 2017a, p. 8). Caritas literacy calls forth the arts and artistry of self and other, and conveys a continually evolving caritas consciousness, moral efficacy, and lifelong journey of self-growth, self-healing, and spiritual practices (Watson, 2008). Caritas literacy is a love of humanity and all living things.

Engaging in this journey means applying the 10 Caritas Processes within the frame of unitary Caring Science. Beyond this it requires ongoing cultivation of caring consciousness and intentionality. From the application of these processes and cultivation of caring consciousness, practitioners become more awake and intentional. They know to pause before entering another's room, read the energetic field, and maintain authentic presence; they see value in *being with* as much as (and at times more than) *doing for*. They integrate caring consciousness with knowledge and skills, expanding and evolving into something more.

Healthcare practitioners rooted in Caring Science develop an expanded quantum worldview related to global principles of human caring and peace. They also acknowledge a deeper "ethic of belonging" (Levinas, 1969; Watson, 2008; Watson, 2017b). This higher consciousness calls for both a local and global commitment to the improvement of quality of life for all human beings (Horton-Deutsch & Rosa, 2017).

Walter's (2017b) theory of emancipatory nursing praxis (ENP) is a hermeneutic-dialectic relational learning process for addressing inequities. In this process, a member of a dominant social group works closely *with* members of an oppressed group to remedy the systematic denial of privilege and power based on social group membership alone. It is presented here as a way to further extend Caring Science and reflective practice toward informed moral praxis and doing. Because Caritas Coaches walk alongside others with universal care and love for all humanity, they are poised for this type of role, being and becoming a social justice ally.

ENP is composed of two contextual categories and four conceptual processes (see Figure 21.2). The two contextual categories are as follows (Walter, 2014; Walter, 2017a):

- **Reflective context:** To become a social justice ally, practitioners move through an inner journey of becoming and awakening, during which they recognize unearned privileges that unjustly benefit them.

- **Relational context:** Through critical reflective dialogue with others, practitioners explore the processes of engaging and transforming, during which they learn to relate to others in more authentic and emancipatory ways. They acquire skills to leverage their privilege, recognizing and challenging oppressive people and systems.

The four conceptual processes are as follows (Walter, 2014; Walter, 2017a):

- **Becoming:** This represents the individual's earliest memories and discernments of social injustice or unfairness. Reflective practices in the becoming process tend to be primarily descriptive. Individuals recount details of experiences in which they witnessed injustice.

- **Awakening:** In this process, individuals identify their role or their place in the larger social context and how that affects the health and well-being of others. Marked by a change in how an individual sees himself or herself in relation to others, awakening allows the individual to question formally held beliefs, attitudes, and assumptions, and to compare them to alternative views of the same situation. During awakening, self-awareness and dialogue are integral to ally development.

- **Engaging:** This refers to the actions and interactions involved in social justice ally work. This dynamic and evolving process actively explores and cultivates the role of ally with the intention of advancing specific transformative goals. The overall intention is to dismantle systems of oppression that create inequity.

- **Transforming:** This represents the motivation for the individual to become a social justice ally. It is viewed as an expansion of consciousness embodying human flourishing, achieving equity, and transforming social relationships.

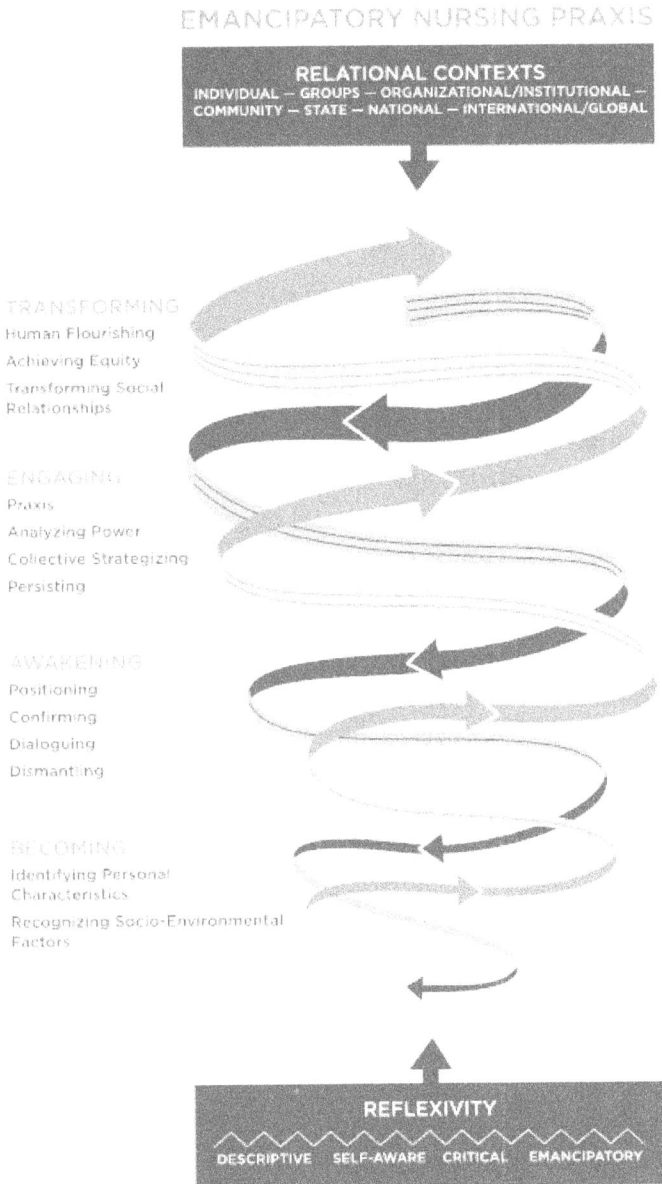

FIGURE 21.2 THE RELATIONSHIP OF THE PROCESSES AND
SUB-PROCESSES OF ENP (WALTER, 2014).

As with caritas, the dynamic energy of ENP occurs within a context of inner and outer reflection. Reflective practices are initially introspective and intrapersonal and evolve to a form of reflexivity firmly grounded in interpersonal interactions and authentic dialogue with others. Reflexive dialogue creates an opportunity to reestablish attitudes and beliefs that generate new meaning in action (praxis) (Walter, 2017b).

The ENP theory contains intricacies beyond the scope of this chapter. Interested readers are directed to the reference list at the end of this chapter to learn more about how this theory can guide informed moral praxis. This process creates a powerful sense of collective agency that empowers practitioners to stand with the marginalized, with the goal of emancipation for both. In all actuality, Caring Science is a social justice model of profound caring. It calls us to become a transformational force and ally for humanity.

FINAL REFLECTIONS

Through the application of Caring Science, the Caritas Coaches who contributed to this book discovered that they had far more influence on their environment than they ever imagined. Each found the capacity to transform their environments for the better. They discovered that the way they approach being, becoming, knowing, and doing affects those around them, and that the responses of those around them in turn affect others. As the effects of small acts delivered with loving-kindness pass from person to person, the impact grows. This can be a source of joy, inspiration, and hope. These small acts are like a stone dropped into still water. They ripple and spread, expanding as they move outward. Integral theory and emancipatory nursing praxis are two frameworks that can further extend this ripple.

The recipient of the love, care, and compassion of a Caritas Coach will likely feel compelled to be more kind and caring toward others; when we feel the effects of positive energy, we are more likely to pass it along. Passing from person to person, a group

movement can eventually transform an entire community, organization, or system. Every transformation, like every ripple, must begin
somewhere. Through the Caritas Coach Education Program, Caritas
Coaches discover their ability to be that point of origin, spreading
loving-kindness to other people, their community, and throughout
the world.

REFERENCES

Dewey, J. (1933). *How we think: A restatement of the relation of reflective thinking to the educative process*. Boston, MA: D. C. Heath and Co.

Horton-Deutsch, S., & Rosa, W. (2017). The role of reflective practice in creating the world we want. In W. Rosa (Ed.), *A new era in global health: Nursing and the United Nations 2030 Sustainable Development Agenda* (pp. 461–474). New York, NY: Springer Publishing Co.

Levinas, E. (1969). *Totality and infinity: An essay on exteriority*. Pittsburgh, PA: Duquesne University Press.

Pesut, D. J. (2017). An introduction to integral philosophy and theory: Implications for quality and safety. In S. Horton-Deutsch & G. D. Sherwood (Eds.), *Reflective practice: Transforming education and improving outcomes* (2nd ed., pp. 315–328). Indianapolis, IN: Sigma Theta Tau International.

Pesut, D. J., Sherwood, G. D., & Horton-Deutsch, S. (2017). Reflecting as a team: Issues to consider in interprofessional practice. In S. Horton-Deutsch & G. D. Sherwood (Eds.), *Reflective practice: Transforming education and improving outcomes* (2nd ed., pp. 331–354). Indianapolis, IN: Sigma Theta Tau International.

Walter, R. W. (2014). A grounded theory study of the critical factors influencing nurse professionals' perceptions of their role in social justice. (Doctoral dissertation.) *PQDT Open*. Retrieved from https://pqdtopen.proquest.com/doc/1836057479.html?FMT=ABS

Walter, R. R. (2017a). Emancipatory nursing praxis: A theory of social justice in nursing. *Advances in Nursing Science, 40*(3), 223–241. doi:10.1097/ANS.0000000000000157

Walter, R. R. (2017b). Emancipatory nursing praxis: Becoming a social justice ally. In S. Horton-Deutsch & G. D. Sherwood (Eds.), *Reflective practice: Transforming education and improving outcomes* (2nd ed., pp. 355–378). Indianapolis, IN: Sigma Theta Tau International.

Watson, J. (2008). *Nursing: The philosophy and science of caring* (rev. ed.). Boulder, CO: University Press of Colorado.

Watson, J. (2017a). *Global advances in human caring literacy*. New York, NY: Springer Publishing Co.

Watson, J. (2017b). Global human caring for a sustainable world. In W. Rosa (Ed.), *A new era in global health: Nursing and the United Nations 2030 Sustainable Development Agenda* (pp. 227–246). New York, NY: Springer Publishing Co.

Watson, J., & Horton-Deutsch, S. (Forthcoming 2018). *Caring science literacy: From caritas to global communitas.* In W. Rosa, S. Horton-Deutsch, & J. Watson (Eds.), *Handbook on caring science*. New York, NY: Springer Publishing Co.

Wilber, K. (2000). *Integral psychology: Consciousness, spirit, psychology, therapy.* Boston, MA: Shambhala Publications.

Wilber, K. (2001). *A theory of everything: An integral vision for business, politics, science and spirituality.* Boston, MA: Shambhala Publications.

Wilber, K. (2005). Introduction to integral theory and practice: IOS basic and the AQAL map. *Journal of Integral Theory and Practice, 1*(1), 1–36.

Wilber, K. (2007). *The integral vision: A very short introduction to the revolutionary integral approach to life, god, the universe, and everything.* Boston, MA: Shambhala Publications.

INDEX

C

equality, 103–108
equanimity, 8, 47, 58
ethical covenants, 6
evolution, 267–268
    as an educator, 69–80
    of Caritas Coaches, 289–302
exhaling, 66. *See also* breathing
    techniques

F

fear, defusing, 64
feedback, 50
finding purpose, 91–92
forgiveness, 58
The Four Agreements: A Practical Guide to Personal Freedom (Ruiz), 271
frame of reference
    exploring the patient's, 132–134
    working from another, 72, 86–88
frameworks, caring, 259–260
Frameworks 4 Change, 70, 73
freedom from ego, 98–100

G

Gadow, Sally, 80
Garabed-Hruska, Jill, 55–67
gentle paradigm, 278
gestalt, 169
Giovannoni, Jill, 147–148
Giovannoni, Joseph, 141–152
global vision (for caritas), 275–285
    art and science of nurse coaching, 277–278
    Billy's caritas journey, 275–285
    caritas literacy, 280–282
    intention, 278–279
    sustenance of self, 282–283
    trust, 279–280
glow, inner, 165–166
God, 6. *See also* source
Goldberg, Lisa, 42–52
gratitude, 58
Griffin, Christine, 95–116

H

Hagle, Heidi J., 153–161
Harry Potter and the Deathly Hallows (Rowling), 254
healers, 149–150. *See also* nursing
healing, 5, 8, 120–121, 131
    caring-healing environments, 154–155
    caring-healing relationships, 163
    caring literacy, 89–90
    environments, 144–146, 262–264
    finding purpose, 91–92
    humanity, 176–177
    informing practice (of caritas), 239–240
    inner glow, 165–166
    Kino's caritas journey, 83–93
    listening with intent, 88–89
    mindfulness, 242–244
    a physician's journey (Jenny's), 237–245
    rituals and symbols, 265–266
    service to others, 84–86
    spirit-to-spirit connections, 241–242
    working from another frame of reference, 86–88
health, 8, 123, 131
healthcare system, 201
heart and emotions, 14
HeartMath, 135, 200, 225–235
HeartMath techniques, 37
honesty environments, 177–179
honor, 6
hope, importance of, 112–114
Horton-Deutsch, Sara, 289–302
human caring, theory of, 4–5
Human Caring Science: A Theory of Nursing (Watson), 167
human caring theory (HCT), 188–190, 191–194
humanism, 6
humanity, healing, 176–177

I

J

K

L

living caritas
authenticity, 110–112
caritas beyond the workplace,
115
Christine's caritas journey,
95–116
environments, 101–103
equality, 103–108
freedom from ego, 98–100
importance of hope, 112–114
service to others, 108–110
Løgstrup, Knud Ejler, 78
love, 137, 142, 201, 208. *See also*
self-love
being grounded in, 118–119
connections, 122–123
healing, 120–121 (*See also*
healing)
narratives, 123–124
Nick's caritas journey, 117–125
transpersonal caring, 121–122
(*See also* transpersonal caring)
loving-kindness, 8, 47, 122–123, 124,
155
becoming a healer, 149–150
being a Caritas Coach, 142–144
forms of knowing, 148
healing environments, 144–146
Joseph's caritas journey, 141–152
maintaining, 146–148
loving others, 164–165

M

mantras, 135
Mathews, Nancy, 225–235
meditation, 60, 63, 92, 227, 228, 259
mentoring, 58
metanoia, definition of, 30
mindfulness, 142, 155, 208, 209–210,
227, 242–244. *See also* meditation
mindfulness-based stress reduction
(MBSR), 34
miracles, 113
models
AQAL (All Quadrants All
Levels), 292–294

care delivery, 191, 199
developing, 65–66
leadership, 71
professional practice models
(PPMs), 191
unitary-transformative caring,
33, 35
moments, caring, 168, 170
Mother Teresa, 160
moving forward, 233–234
multidimensionality of being, 252–
253

N

narratives, 123–124
Nightingale, Florence, 178, 198, 262
nonjudgmental attitudes, 135
nurse coaching, art and science of,
277–278
Nurse Coach Practice Competencies,
15–23
nurse educators
Lisa's caritas journey, 42–52
philosophies for, 41–53
nurses
helping to find their voice, 35–36
learning path of, 173–183
recruitment, 191–194
nursing
service to others, 85
skills, 9
*Nursing: The Philosophy and Science
of Caring* (Watson), 5, 188, 241
nurturing
compassion, 63
self, 58–59

O

objectives, 10
Okakura (1919), 49
Oman, Kathleen S., 69–80
open hearts, 129. *See also* open minds
open minds, 78, 129–140

Y–Z

www.ingramcontent.com/pod-product-compliance
Lightning Source LLC
Chambersburg PA
CBHW061622220326
41598CB00026BA/3844